COOKING FOR CHEMO... AND AFTER!

Second Edition
Written By Chef Ryan Callahan

Edited By Jessie Callahan
Published By Callahan Publishing
ISBN: 9781726291958

Written, Edited, and Produced in the USA
Cooking for Chemo... and After! Second Edition printed October 2018
Cooking for Chemo... and After! Version 1.5 printed July 2016
Cooking for Chemo... and After! First Edition printed June 2015

Visit Our Websites:
CookingForChemo.org
ChefRyanCallahan.com
CallahanPublishing.com

Follow Chef Ryan Online:
Instagram: @chef_ryan_callahan
Twitter: @cookingforchemo

TABLE OF CONTENTS

INTRODUCTION

Everyone is different. If there is nothing else that you take from this book, this is the single most important idea that you can take with you. Because everyone is different, not every solution is as simple as one size fits all. Because of this, you will have to do much leg work and at home participation to adapt these techniques that I will teach you to your own personal situation.

Cancer is not a battle. It is a war. You must constantly work at beating it without fatigue or tiring out. If you are not willing to run the marathon, you can not beat cancer. With that being said, in this book you will learn how to adjust your cooking to accommodate for eating related chemotherapy side effects. Through this process I will do my best to equip you with the weapons and tools needed to win the war against starvation.

20-50% of all cancer related deaths are due to systematic starvation *(cachexia)*. This shockingly high figure is even higher in terminal cancer patients with starvation accounting for 80% of cancer related deaths. We believe that learning how to cook at home, and learning how to adjust your cooking for the taste and smell changes that occur during cancer treatment, can help prevent starvation. Learning how to cook, in addition to working with your dietitian and oncologist to make certain you are getting the proper nutrients that your body needs to survive, is the key to help prevent starvation. By understanding these taste changes, you are better equipped to communicate your needs and your preferences to your dietitian, who can then help you fill in any gaps in your nutrition. It really is two fold, you must want to succeed and be willing to do or learn whatever is necessary to succeed.

Let's begin with the basics. What is this book? *Cooking for Chemo ...and After!* is a guide book that will give you a greater understanding of what a person going through chemotherapy is dealing with when it comes to eating related side effects. This book, as previously stated, requires effort on the part of the reader to learn culinary concepts, try them at home, and learn how to change your own perception of food and flavor in the process. The beginning of this book is written to teach you the information that you need to know BEFORE you ever set foot in the kitchen. The recipes at the end of the book are simply recipes that worked for my mom and other cancer patients that I have worked with in the past. They are NOT a nutritional guide. They are NOT a cure for cancer. They are NOT for everyone. The recipes are a guideline to help you understand how I design recipes to accommodate for eating related side effects like nausea, metallic taste, and loss of appetite.

This is where you the reader come in. By learning the culinary theories in the front half of this book, you will be able to understand how to change ANY recipe to suit your needs and dietary preferences. A perfect example of this is an acquaintance of mine who is a vegan. She makes French onion soup, but omits beef broth and cheese by replacing them with a porcini mushroom broth and a vegan cheese. She still follows the Roundness of Flavor chart when she seasons. As a result, it is so close to authentic French onion soup that the difference in flavor is undetectable.

This above concept is one of the many concepts you will learn in this book. What you will learn in this book is the following:

1. How to understand the relationship between food, flavor, and flavor perception.

2. How to change flavors using Roundness of Flavor.

3. How to understand the changes in flavor perception that occur as a result of cancer treatments.

4. How to combat and accommodate for the following side effects: loss of appetite, nausea, metallic taste, mouth sores, and difficulty chewing and swallowing.

5. What solutions to eating related side effects work and do not work.

6. What to keep in mind BEFORE cooking for someone with cancer.

7. Comfort food is subjective to life experience.

8. Basic nutritional information.

9. Basic meal planning.

10. Grocery shopping on a budget.

11. Food safety and sanitation rules.

After these 11 very important concepts are discussed, there is an entire section of the book dedicated to recipes that will help you focus your attempts at cooking and eating. The recipe sections are ordered from heaviest weighted foods to lightest weighted foods and in alphabetical order within their own sections. What we mean by weight is residue of flavor they leave in your mouth and heaviness in your stomach after eating. We have found that the heavier recipes are fine for early treatment and the lighter recipes are better for severe side effects and later in treatment.

How do I use this book?

Using this book is very easy. You begin by reading the pages in the front sequentially in numerical order until you reach the recipe sections. After you reach the recipe sections, pick recipes that sound appealing to the cancer patient and begin cooking. This is where the built in tasting journals come into play. As they taste each recipe, make notes inside of the tasting journal pages to help you refine your culinary technique to fall in line with the cancer patients preferences. Be forewarned though, a cancer patients preferences change with treatment, time, what medications they are on, and the concentrations of those medications in their body. It's a bit like trying to hit a bulls-eye a mile away, while riding a horse across a ships deck in rough seas. It is very difficult, but it can be done.

Do not skip ahead in the book. Every section builds on the previous section just like a text book. These sections are laid out so that you may come back to them and re-read them as a refresher course.

Why did I write this book?

I wrote this book because of my personal connection to cancer. Both of my grandfathers died from cancer as did my best friend in college. In the spring of 2013, my mother was diagnosed with HER2+ breast cancer and this began my year as a full time caregiver. With my previous experience with cancer and chemotherapy, I knew that an inability to eat and metallic taste was on the menu for my mother. What I did not know about was mouth sores, nausea, and a general disinterest in food. All of these side effects combined gave me a very difficult challenge while trying to make my mothers cancer journey as easy as possible.

It was during this time as a caregiver that I discovered the breakthroughs that I now include in my books that help cancer patients eat again. For a more a detailed story, please see our website: *cookingforchemo.org*

Why do you need this book?

You need this book because nobody beats cancer alone. It is through the help of friends, family, and many qualified professionals that we are able to beat cancer. For many people, this book becomes a life line to sanity and humanity. This is because metallic tastes and constant nausea can break down your hope and will power to fight. We want to give these back to you. What fills your heart with love faster than a warm belly, laughter, and loved ones?

Very specifically, we are going to teach you in this book everything you need to know to combat the most common eating related chemotherapy side effects. This will empower you to work with your dietitian and oncologist to get the nutrients your body needs to win. And if that wasn't enough, we are also going to teach you a life long skill that will make you the hit of every party, outing, and family get together. Let me tell ya something. Knowing how to cook is a bit like being the only person in your family that owns a pick up truck *(lorry)*. Everyone is going to want to use your services all the time.

This book assumes that you have a very minimal grasp on basic culinary techniques. It assumes you are familiar with words like sauté, stir fry, chop, mince, and much more. If you are brand new to cooking, be not afraid as I have already written a fun, friendly cookbook that actually teaches you how to cook. I would recommend picking up a copy of my book, *Chef Ryan's How-to Cook Cookbook* as a supplementary resource to this book. You can find this book via my personal website: *chefryancallahan.com*

With all that being said, let's get excited and prepared to learn everything you need to know about *Cooking for Chemo*!

PART 1: FOUNDATIONS OF COOKING FOR CHEMO

LESSON 1: UNDERSTANDING THE EATING EXPERIENCE

The very first idea you must understand when cooking for someone undergoing chemotherapy treatments is how flavors and the eating experience are perceived. In my experience, I have learned that it is not the flavors of the foods that cancer patients eat but their *perception of these foods* that have changed. Chemotherapy plays havoc on the entirety of your body, not just the cancer cells it is targeting. This is why your hair falls out, your skin gets sores, and your nails become brittle. The same effects can also be felt on all of your sensory organs as well.

Let's discuss a simple example. Imagine if you will, that a grilled chicken breast covered in a sweet tangy barbecue sauce is your favorite dish of all time. Now, imagine it is being served to you and you are extremely hungry. The smell, sight, and taste of that grilled chicken will be one of the greatest pleasures of your life. Now imagine that same situation, but you had far too many cocktails last night and are dizzy, nauseous, and feel like you are going to throw up. What is the smell and sight of that chicken going to do to you in that situation? Is that grilled chicken going to be one of the greatest pleasures of your life? Or will it be one of your greatest displeasures? The answer is very simple. The smell of that chicken breast alone will make your nausea even worse than it was before. Any hunger that you had will dissipate and you will probably want to go right back to bed.

Notice how in our simple example the chicken breast has not changed, but our *perception* of it has. This is what is happening to everyone undergoing chemotherapy treatments. It is even more true if you are on extremely high doses of chemotherapy. So, from this point forward, always keep this idea in mind.

"It is not what food tastes like to the caregiver. It is what food tastes like to the patient."

In this lesson, I am going to elaborate on this idea and help you to understand the relationship between the perception of food and its resulting flavor. I am also going to teach you how you perceive food with all of your senses.

Defining Your Senses

By conventional definition, you possess, or should possess, 5 distinct senses. They are taste, touch, smell, sight, and sound. These conventional 5 senses are how you perceive the world. But during the eating experience, there is a sixth sense that comes into play. It is called memory association. No. The sixth sense is not a super power, but it gives your present experiences historical and learned context. Let's discuss each sense and how it comes into play during the eating experience.

Taste
Everyone knows taste and food go together. As a matter of fact, we often ask each other while eating,

"how does it taste?" Your sense of taste is a sense that only operates by physical contact with the item that is being perceived. Your tongue is where your sense of taste is located and food and liquids have to physically touch the taste receptors located on your tongue to be perceived. Your sense of taste is limited to only 5 experiences. They are:

salty

savory

spicy

sour

sweet

We will discuss these 5 flavors, in detail, later in this book.

During chemotherapy treatments, each one of these flavors can change in intensity and sensitivity. This causes a misalignment of understanding what foods are supposed to taste like and what they currently taste like. Instead of a cheeseburger tasting like a cheeseburger to you, it could in theory, taste like eggplant parmesan. This later part, has more to do with memory association coming into play, which you will learn about in just a moment.

Smell

Your sense of smell is the first of your senses that allows you to perceive an object or item from a distance. Virtually all objects in the world have some sort of smell. Contrary to popular belief, your sense of smell is actually your most complex and advanced sense. You can perceive over a trillion unique scents and distinguish them individually from each other. Interestingly, your sense of smell is also your strongest sense tied to memory. As a result, the whiff of something like cologne can immediately draw up memories of your grandfather. If you really close your eyes and concentrate, you will notice that as you think of these memories, you can actually re-smell the events in your mind as if they were happening right now.

For example, let us pretend that you have a pot roast simmering in a slow cooker. Your house is filled with the smell of pot roast. As a result, it smells so good you can taste it, right? Wrong. You don't actually taste the pot roast just from smelling it. But, you are using your sense of smell to experience the flavor for you. The most complicated flavors that you will experience are generated not by your tongue's interaction with your food, but with your nose's interaction with your food.

Another thing you absolutely must know is the concept of pungency. Pungency is simply defined as how powerful the smell of an item is. For example, roses have a light smell and are not very pungent. But, old fish is very pungent and will have an off-putting smell. Some would say that smell is stinky. To differentiate, pungency describes the *quantity* or concentration of odors. Where as stinky describes the *quality* of odors. Understanding the variations in the strength of pungency is something you will learn to develop as time goes on and as you become more proficient with your cooking techniques. Smell is also strongly tied to the side effect nausea and we will discuss this in greater detail later in this book.

Touch

Your sense of touch is another sense where proximity and physical contact are required. Your sense of touch exists inside of the skin cells that cover your body. When you physically press your skin against another object, you perceive that it is there. Your sense of touch is also connected to your perception of pain. With chemotherapy treatments, this often manifests itself in the form of mouth sores. Your sense of touch manifests itself in the perception of food textures.

Food texture is extremely important to consider for 3 reasons:

1. By varying the texture, you can completely change the character of the dish.
2. Many people have texture aversions, not necessarily taste aversions.
3. Mouth sores create sensitivity to abrasive textures, spicy foods, and to foods that are hot in temperature.

A perfect example of a texture aversion is with mushrooms. Most people love the flavor and smell of sautéed mushrooms. But because of their slimy texture, many people avoid them in entirety. The solution to this is simply to finely dice the mushrooms so that the flavor is still there but the texture has changed into something that more people will find palatable.

Texture defines the quality of dishes and helps the person eating the dish decide their emotional response to the dish based solely on the texture. Chicken and dumplings, like most comfort foods, has a very soft and soupy texture from hours of slow cooking. On the other hand, uncooked raw vegetables have a crisp and firm texture. This crisp texture imparts a feeling of freshness and a pleasing bite that is especially great for snacking.

When cooking, you want to always take texture into consideration when you are creating a dish. This helps influence the emotional state of the person who is eating the food. You want to use texture to tell your diner how to feel about your dish. This is how texture ties into memory association.

Sight

This is your second sense that allows you to perceive objects from a distance. Light bounces off of an object, enters your eyes, and you then perceive the object. Even though humans are eye dominant, we can only perceive a few million actual colors. But because we are sight dominant, we use sight to distinguish good and bad, pleasant and unpleasant, and even eating choices. Why do you think there are pictures on restaurant menus? Sight comes into play in the chemotherapy experience by helping to build or diminish an appetite from a distance.

Because humans are extremely visually influenced, a dish can be cast aside simply by looking at the dish. Look at any culinary competition on the television. The judges will always comment on the visual appeal and presentation of the dishes that they have been presented before they even take a bite. It is important to use this knowledge that sight influences a persons eating habits before we begin cooking so that we can cater everything we cook to the preferences of those we are cooking for.

Using lots of fresh vegetables in our cooking is not only a great source of nutrition, but is also wonderful to create visually appealing dishes. One of my favorite dishes is called, cacio e pepe. This dish is very simple in the fact that it is spaghetti noodles, pecorino romano, and black pepper. It tastes wonderful, but is visually very unappealing. On the other hand, a summer salad with cucumber, grape tomatoes, red onions, Kalamata olives, and feta cheese creates a visually striking dish. Once you see a picture of it, you are immediately hungry and want to eat that salad.

By using bright and varied color inside of our dishes, it allows us to create appetizing dishes before they even hit the table.

Sound

Your sense of hearing is your third sense that allows you to process information from a distance. Very simply, vibrations in the air actuate the mechanical parts of your inner ear and transmit the sound to your brain in a way that you can interpret. Sound is how we process conversations, music, and ambient noises. Sound is also how we process certain textures like "crunchy."

Sound comes into play in 3 different, but 3 very important ways:

1. There is, of course, the auditory experience of the actual eating experience.

   For example, you slurp soup, you crunch chips, and you hear the clinking and clanking of tableware to indicate that people are eating.

2. By using our sense of sound during the actual cooking process, we can begin to attune our senses to perceive the condition of the doneness of food, with out visually seeing the cooking process.

   For example, water makes a boiling sound, sautéing makes a crackling popping sound, grilling makes a searing sound. When you hear the water boiling, you know that it's time to drop the noodles into the water to cook them. When properly sautéing something, you can train your ear to listen to the sizzling sound of the water escaping the food product to know if the food has been sufficiently sautéed and whether it is time to flip it. The searing sound of steak on a grill is actually the sound of moisture escaping from the meat. The louder the searing sound is, the faster it is occurring, and therefore you can tell how hot your grill is. Once you stop hearing sizzling or searing sounds, you know that the moisture has been completely cooked out of your food, which is not always ideal.

But by learning the sounds inside of the cooking process, you may observe new information with a far underutilized sense.

3. When you hear the sounds of cooking, you can begin to become hungry.

You don't have to smell, see, or taste food to know that there is food cooking. The rhythmic clanging of a sauté pan and the sizzling sound of sautéing mushrooms is enough to tell someone that there is something delicious happening in the kitchen. This becomes an association when these actions are followed by the ingestion of food.

When I was my mothers caregiver, I always did 2 things before I would feed her:

1. I would play old crooner music, so that she would know that I was cooking.
2. I would always begin by sautéing something delicious in a sauté pan.

Over time, she began to associate the sounds of cooking and old crooner music with delicious food and learned that it was an appropriate time to be hungry. Now, we will learn more about memory association and how it plays into the 5 senses.

Memory Association

These first 5 senses are constantly feeding information into your brain. This information is recorded live and then your brain passes this information through a series of conditional filters, one of which compares present situations to past situations. These past situations, or "memories," find similar patterns to give a present day situation learned historical context and these contexts become associations. I am sure this sounds a little complicated, but you do this naturally and without having to consciously think about it all the time.

Memory association helps you to make decisions quicker by prejudicing your decisions towards familiar and successful choices in the past. Think of it like this, "if X worked in the past, X should work today." As a chef, you must break yourself out of certain eating and association cycles so that you may grow in experience and understanding of different cuisines and cultures. Every time you learn something new or taste a new food that information is incorporated into your database and helps you to make better, more informed, and new decisions.

Memory association comes into play during the eating experience by helping you decide what foods and drinks you would like to ingest. This becomes problematic during cancer treatment because your input data from your senses does not match the historical data to which it has been referenced. This can cause frustration, disinterest in food, and loss of appetite.

Now that you understand the basics of how each sense functions, we can dive into flavor, the eating experience, and how chemo treatments change your eating experience.

Food For Thought
Think about what you just learned and how it applies to your situation. Ask yourself these questions.

1. What sense(s) did you not realize were part of the eating experience?

2. Which sense(s) do you rely on the most?

LESSON 2: THE 5 FLAVORS

Flavor is a tricky and complicated concept. It is made up of many different aspects of senses as well as senses in their entirety. Let's start with the basics of the tongue. The human tongue only tastes a few basic flavors. This is actually such a controversial subject that it is still hotly debated whether or not certain flavors constitute tasting or just a secondary experience. The most commonly accepted flavors that your tongue tastes are: salty, savory, sour, bitter, and sweet. I like to add spicy to this list as well, seeing as you experience spicy on your tongue just like the other flavors. I don't consider bitter to be a flavor, but I consider it to be a survival mechanism. Therefore, I do not include it in the 5 flavors. So for simplicity—and for our sanity—we will say that the following are the flavors that you actually taste with your tongue: salty, savory, spicy, sour, and sweet.

This information is important to know because your perception of the 5 flavors changes during chemotherapy treatments. As I had said in the previous lesson, your historical knowledge of each flavor does not line up with your current perception of the experience of each flavor.

So, we must begin first by:

1. Understanding what each flavor actually tastes like in its raw essence.
2. We must re-learn what these flavors taste like to the cancer patient today.

The following exercise will help both caregivers and patients understand the differences between each flavor and how their sense of taste *(palate)* has shifted due to chemotherapy treatments. Often, you will hear the word "palate." The word in this context means your personal taste preferences.

So, let's have some fun at home and learn what role your tongue plays in experiencing flavor. We're going to do an experiment tasting the 5 flavors through different seasonings and truly experiencing them for the first time. In the following at home activity, you will taste the 5 flavors that your tongue perceives as a raw, singular flavor with no interference from outside flavors or senses.

At Home Activity - Tasting the Five Flavors

Ingredients Needed:
1 tsp. kosher salt
1 tsp. soy sauce or MSG
1 tsp. red pepper, black pepper, or cayenne pepper
1 tsp. red wine vinegar, lemon juice, or lime juice
1 tsp. granulated white table sugar or honey
a glass of water for rinsing

Directions:
First, wash and dry your hands to avoid cross-contamination. Using a series of small containers, place each of the above ingredients into their own separate containers. Make certain none of the seasonings are mixed with other seasonings. Before you taste each one, pinch your nose to stop the sensation of smell from becoming involved. This is so that you can finally taste something purely with your tongue and not with your sense of smell. Now, using the tip of your finger, taste each one individually. Wash your mouth out and fingers off with water before trying the next ingredient.

Using the basic senses we just described, fill in the blank with what each ingredient tastes like to you.

At Home Activity: Taste the 5 Flavors Chart

Ingredient	Taste of Ingredient
kosher salt	
soy sauce	
MSG	
red pepper, black pepper, or cayenne pepper	
red wine vinegar	
lemon juice or lime juice	
granulated white sugar or honey	

Did you notice how the flavors that you associate with each item vary greatly from what you think of in your mind verses what the actual flavor is inside of your mouth? Since salt mostly activates in the front portion of your tongue, those are the taste receptors that come alive when you taste it. Savory perception is mostly located in the back of your tongue. It often feels like a very subtle and muted flavor. Knowing where the location of each flavor sense exists isn't the important part of this lesson. It is in knowing that your tongue has dedicated flavor receptors for each flavor and that they are not mixed in together evenly. This should be your first ah-ha moment of this book. You have just begun to discover how each part of your body comes into play when you perceive flavor.

Now, let's do this experiment again. But this time, describe how your mouth physically feels after each item.

At Home Activity: Mouth Feel of Flavor Chart

Ingredient	How it FEELS In Your Mouth
kosher salt	
soy sauce	
MSG	
red pepper, black pepper or cayenne pepper	
red wine vinegar	
lemon juice or lime juice	
granulated white sugar or honey	

So why does the way food feels in your mouth matter? The reason you need to know how something feels in your mouth when cooking has to do with the concept of weight. *Weight* is the sensation of food in your mouth. A dish's weight can be anywhere from heavy to light just like all physical objects. This is important because seasonal cooking relies very heavily on the concept of weight.

For example, winter dishes like shepherd's pie tend to be very heavy in weight. It is filled with proteins, starches, and fats. It generally causes a heavy feeling in your stomach and in your mouth during and after eating. On the other hand, a nice Greek salad with vinaigrette dressing, and the whole nine yards of fresh ingredients in it, is a perfect example of a lightly weighted summer dish. The large amount of calories from complex animal fats is one of the many reasons the shepherd's pie feels heavier in weight than the Greek salad. We will talk more about the concept of "weight" in the upcoming lessons.

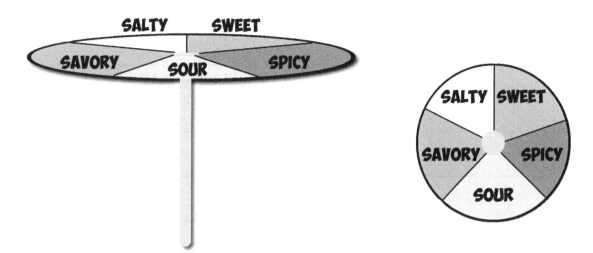

Balancing The Five Flavors

When a chef cooks, what he is trying to do is bring out the fullness of flavor, or Roundness of Flavor. This brings us to our next lesson.

Think about the results of our sensory perception test and what you know these flavors to be. Now take a look at the chart above for a great visual representation of what I call, Roundness of Flavor.

Imagine the circular dish above is mounted on a thin piece of metal so that it acts as a scale. As you apply weight to any category, like salty, the dish will tip toward the salty side. As you place each flavor on the dish, it will lean from side to side, eventually balancing out. What you want to do is weigh out the proper amounts of flavor onto this imaginary dish so that the dish doesn't topple over and become one-sided.

Cooking is about balance, harmony, and pulling the natural flavors out of your ingredients. All food items that you eat have their own natural flavors and will pre-stack the weight of the dish. As we add items to our meals, we need to be conscious of their natural flavors and how they will make the dish balance.

To be blunt, there is simply no way to teach someone to cook without physically doing it. You can learn many other disciplines simply by reading about it. But, cooking is both art and science. Just like you can never truly create great works of art simply by looking at Vincent Van Gogh's paintings. You will never develop the physical techniques of the intricacies inherent inside of the brush strokes to capture the delicateness of color. Such is the same with great food. Learning how to cook is exactly like this. You must try and fail and try and fail until you learn how things work and why. Just like the yoga master refers to the art of yoga as "my practice," so must we take this same approach toward cooking. It is an art that you will continually become greater at every day, every week, and every year. You will learn and grow just like a tree until your roots run so far into the ground that you are an immovable object with years of strength and experience to pull from. So it is with this mind-set, we will continue to move forward so that we may practice and learn.

What I would like to explain about Roundness of Flavor is that I actually developed this cooking technique to specifically help my mother while she was going through cancer treatments. But, Roundness of Flavor isn't just for cancer patients. It is also an incredibly effective and fool-proof system for progressively and accurately seasoning your food so that it turns out nearly perfect every single time.

Below is the method I follow while creating my own Roundness of Flavor. I do this with every single dish, no matter how simple or how complex. This is the creating flavor part of Roundness of Flavor. When I season dishes, I always season them in the following order:

1. salty
2. savory
3. spicy
4. sour
5. sweet

Understanding the Five Flavors

Salty

Salty is the most basic flavor. It is also the most powerful. It amplifies all other flavors. We start with salty to bring out the naturally occurring flavors in the dish. If we did this flavor later, it could overpower the rest of the dish. Adding salt late in the cooking process could make the flavors too aggressive. On the other hand, food without salt of any kind is extremely bland. If you can not have salt because of sodium, consider using a salt substitute. Salt is also one of the flavors that you cannot correct if you add too much. If you place too much salt in a dish, it is simply ruined and you have to start over.

Examples of salty items: kosher salt, sea salt, soy sauce, and hard cheeses like parmesan.

Savory

I always season savory second because it is the least pronounced of all the flavors. *But, it is the most important.* The reason it is so important is because it gives you that sense of deliciousness and satisfaction that comes from a home-cooked meal. Savory is the fullness of taste. It is the sense of warmth that you get when eating a protein filled item. Savory is actually activated by the presence of salty flavor. This is the reason why a steak without salt is extremely bland. But if you add a light pinch of salt, it makes the steak taste like a flavor explosion. There are many ways to create a savory flavor, whether it is simply adding savory ingredients or using heat to brown your meats and vegetables. Browning these items makes them naturally more savory as well.

Examples of savory items: soy sauce, MSG, anchovies, green tea, mushrooms, tomatoes, and red wine.

Spicy

Spicy comes third because it is our second amplifying flavor. It is the ingredient that fills our warmth portion of the dish. I also season with spicy third because it is the easiest to counter-act by adding more vinegar to balance out the spicy. Please remember that just because you are adding a touch of spicy to a dish does not mean that the dish will necessarily be spicy. Great cooking always encompasses a bit of an imperceptible spicy note that just adds a fuller body. So never feel guilty adding a little bit of spicy to your dishes, especially in amounts that a person cannot detect. To add ingredients that a person cannot name or quite put their finger on is the hallmark of a great chef.

Examples of spicy items: black pepper, cayenne pepper, red pepper flakes, chilies, and many more.

Sour

Sour comes fourth because it is the lightener. Everything we have put into our dishes so far has added breadth, fullness, and warmth. Now, we add complexity. Sour brings freshness that you cannot get through any other means. It removes the physical weight of a dish, similar to how moon boots remove the feeling of weight from your body.

Sour is an amazing flavor that is far underutilized. It can make you feel as if you were eating the freshest, lightest fruit salad in the world. But when applied too heavily and too liberally, it can make your mouth pucker and eyes water. With a masterful hand, sour can be applied in just the right amounts to give heavy dishes a light feeling in your mouth. It can also remove the spiciness while amplifying the flavor of chilies. And, it can cleanse the palate and bring delight to any person who wields it. In my opinion, mastery of sour is another hallmark of a great chef.

Sour is also the primary activator in the palate cleansing technique that we will learn shortly. Palate cleansing is important to know as it is the primary remover of metallic tastes.

Examples of sour items: red vinegar, red wine vinegar, apple cider vinegar, balsamic vinegar, rice wine vinegar, orange juice, lime juice, lemon juice, and pickle brine.

Sweet
Sweet comes last because it is the great balancer. Sweet activates the pleasure centers of your brain and gets you really excited about eating whatever it is you are eating. Sweet can cover many mistakes when cooking and should be used last because it creates our final piece of complex flavoring.

Chinese cooks have a saying that sugar always follows vinegar. This is because sour needs a balancer just like the idea of yin and yang. When yin gets out of control, it needs yang to balance. The philosophy is all about finding the balance between the two. The same is true for fire and water. Fire keeps water in check by boiling it. And water keeps fire in check by keeping it from getting too hot and consuming everything around it. If you have too much fire, everything gets burned. If you have too much water, the passion and the drive is drowned out. The same is true for sour and sweet. You must keep the two in balance at all times. Sweet also allows you to remove or cover the acidity of a dish. Hence, why most people will add a healthy pour of sugar to their marinara sauce.

Sweet is a place where I get a lot of irrational feedback. I am not telling you to pour a pound of sugar into your meals or eat nothing but refined sugars. What I am explaining to you here is that sweetness balances out the dish. It is one of your 5 fundamental flavors. And, it must be mastered and utilized to truly cook like a great chef. A lot of people are afraid of sugar because somebody offhandedly said to them once that people need to eat less sugar.

What those people were trying to actually express was that most people ingest too much candy, sweets, junk food, soft drinks, etc. When you take control of your food and cook every meal at home, you are not going to end up eating too much sugar simply because the nature of cooking at home does not make it easy to overload yourself on sugars. What overloads you on sugar is eating a pint of ice cream, followed by drinking 2 liters of soda, and eating a handful of hard candies to finish off the meal. Remember all things in moderation.

Sugar is actually the basic energy that your body uses to fuel itself. The reason your body is hot is because your body is regularly combusting sugars inside of your cells to regulate your body temperature. When there is too much sugar, your body converts it for long term storage into fat cells which is how your metabolic process works. This is why if you eat too much sugar, you gain weight. If you eat too little sugar, you loose weight. The energy inside of food is measured in calories, which is why all of our food labels are labeled with the amount of calories that are contained within the food. This is so that you can empower yourself to make decisions on how many calories you need to fuel your body. It's not scary. It's science.

Sweet can be sourced from the following: raw granulated sugar, brown sugar, fruit juices, honey, and an innumerable amount of places.

I follow the salty, savory, spicy, sour, sweet method because my experience has taught me that this is how you should season. It takes into account many different theories, styles, and cultures perspectives on cooking. As I stated previously, I have found that cooking is both art and science. It is a beautiful alchemy that encompasses so much of the human spirit, life experience, culture, memories, and the soul; that it is like an art. The simple whiff of your favorite dish can transport you to places and times that you didn't even remember existed. It can pull emotions so deep that you didn't even know you had. *This is the art of cooking.*

Remember that pulling those memories up is called memory association. We must re-learn our associations when we are *Cooking for Chemo*. I will discuss more on this topic in later lessons.

To bring it all around, the reason I season in this method is two fold. Years of experience show me scientifically that this is the right way to season. And, years of artistic endeavor also support this method.

Here are some flavor charts that will help you adjust specific flavors in your dishes. You may want to earmark or post a sticky note on this page. It is a super helpful reference to have on hand while you are cooking, especially while you are first learning.

Basic Flavors Chart: Where to find each flavor in its raw essence

Flavor Order	Where to Find
salty *(amplifier)*	kosher salt, table salt, seasoned salt, soy sauce
savory *(fullness)*	MSG, anchovies, kelp, red wine, green tea, soy sauce, bay leaves, meats, mushrooms
spicy *(amplifier)*	red pepper, cayenne pepper, black pepper, hot sauce
sour *(lightener)*	red wine vinegar, rice vinegar, red vinegar, fermented foods, pickles
sweet *(balancer)*	sugar, brown sugar, molasses, syrup, fruits, honey

Roundness of Flavor Chart: How to correct flavor in a dish

Problem	Solution
dish is bland/not savory	add salt and MSG or soy sauce
dish has no heat	add red pepper or cayenne
dish is too spicy	add red wine vinegar
dish feels heavy in my mouth	add red wine vinegar for a palate cleanser
dish is bitter/sour	add sugar *(remember: sugar follows vinegar)*
dish is too sweet	add red wine vinegar
dish has no pizzazz/aromatic quality	add more herbs or spices

One last thing, when you are trying to correct a dish, always add seasonings in small increments. You don't want to over-correct the dish and have to start over. Let's practice proper seasoning order and increments in the following at home activity.

At Home Activity: Seasoning a Broth Using the Five Flavors

Ingredients Needed:

1 tbsp. kosher salt

1 tbsp. soy sauce or MSG

1 tbsp. red pepper, black pepper, or cayenne pepper

1 tbsp. red wine vinegar

1 tbsp. granulated white table sugar

1 c. chicken or vegetable broth

Directions:

In a small sauce pan, heat broth over medium heat until broth begins to boil.

Remove pan from heat and taste using a clean spoon. CAUTION! The broth will be extremely hot. Pinch your nose while tasting the broth to prevent your sense of smell from becoming involved. After tasting the broth, take notes on the flavor of the broth using the lines that are provided on the next page.

Now, slowly add each of the 5 basic flavors, one at a time, in very small increments. Do not add the full amounts as called for by the ingredient list. Stir thoroughly to dissolve the seasoning completely. Add one at a time and taste after adding each individual flavor. Make notes using the chart on the next page after you stir in each individual flavor.

Start with salty, and move linearly through each flavor, as I have prescribed. Taste in between each flavor to experience and understand how the flavor of the broth changes in between each seasoning. Makes notes on the lines indicating what each flavor did for the broth. After seasoning with all five flavors, adjust the broth to your specific flavor preferences as needed. Did you like it a little more spicy? Add more black pepper. Did you like the broth a little lighter? Add more red wine vinegar.

This exercise helps both the caregiver and the cancer patient understand how flavors develop inside of a real food item and helps both parties to understand the persons preferences.

Make notes about how the flavor of the broth changed as you seasoned it here:

Before seasoning:
After salt:
After MSG:
After black pepper:
After red wine vinegar:
After sugar:

Food For Thought

Think about what you just learned and how it applies to your situation. Ask yourself these questions.

1. How did the broth change as you adjusted the seasoning?

2. Do the 5 flavors taste like you thought they tasted?

3. What flavor is your favorite?

4. What flavor is your least favorite?

5. How will you apply this information in your cooking?

LESSON 3:
MIXNG THE FLAVORS

Now that we have a basic understanding of the 5 flavors as they exist independently, we now need to discuss the interactions that 2 or more flavors have while interacting simultaneously.

Secondary Flavor Senses

Now as we are trying to build our Roundness of Flavor, it is important to keep in mind one other thing. Sometimes, we are trying to construct a dish that specifically bolsters one or more flavor elements.

Two examples of this would be:

1. buffalo style chicken wings and
2. sweet and sour chicken

These are examples of dishes where the end goal would not necessarily be to make the flavors round and equal, but to use the other flavors to compliment the primary flavor of spicy or sweet and sour.

Let's take the example of buffalo style chicken wings and deconstruct the flavor profile of a common recipe. For those of you who aren't familiar with buffalo style chicken wings, they are bone-in chicken wings. These are *(preferably)* deep-fried, then covered in a spicy, tangy sauce.

Usually the sauce is made like this:
8 ounces *[235 ml]* Frank's Red Hot Sauce + 8 ounces *[225 grams]* melted butter *(2 sticks)*.

That gives the wings a creamy, spicy, and tangy sauce.

The 2 questions we need to ask ourselves:

1. What ingredients give the wings a creamy, spicy, and tangy flavor?

The hot sauce is primarily constructed of cayenne peppers that have been infused into a vinegar based solution. Butter tends to have a sweet and savory taste to it. So when you combine hot sauce and butter, you get sweet and savory from the butter, spicy from the chilies, and sour from the vinegar in the sauce.

In the grand scheme, where does this new tangy flavor come into play? Tangy comes from the application of both sour and sweet taste buds at the same time. What is happening in your mouth is that the sour flavor is telling your brain that this food is dry and astringent which causes your mouth to salivate more. But, the sweet flavor is activating the pleasure centers of your brain filling you with endorphins that tell your brain, "This is great! Eat more!" This is also known as the sweet and sour effect.

The same confusing experience can be demonstrated by grasping two pipes filled with water. If one has cold water and the other warm water, it will confuse the sensory nerves in your hands and tell your brain "Danger! This is hot!" Even though the pipes are not hot, your brain believes it is in danger and kicks your survival reflexes in to prevent further potential skin damage. In this same way, the application of both sweet and sour taste receptors confuses your brain causing both pleasure and pain.

Tangy is a perfect example of a secondary flavor sense in action. These secondary flavor senses help to create the complex flavors that we experience when we eat everyday foods.

A secondary flavor sense is only considered secondary when two specific flavors are activated.

For example, if we added MSG *(savory)* to our buffalo wing sauce, causing the tangy flavor to be overwhelmed, we would no longer consider it a secondary flavor but a blended, complimentary flavor.

2. How can we improve on the flavor of a common recipe?

One of the things we can do to improve this chicken wing recipe is we can start by adding salt. When salt is added to savory flavors, it generates a secondary flavor sense I call amplified savory.

The single most important concept in seasoning is that both salty and spicy are flavor amplifiers. What this means is that anything you add salt or spiciness to is going to amplify the flavors of the food already present. Unless you add them in such amounts that they overwhelm the already existing flavors to become the dominant flavors of the dish. Interestingly, the only two flavors that are commonly eaten in western cooking without other complimentary flavors are sweet and savory. Think of hard candies or a big hunk of meat right off the grill. These items are still generally improved with the addition of a little salt, but can very commonly be eaten without.

What else could we add to chicken wings to improve them? We could add black pepper for aromatics and a different type of spicy. *(Yes, each source of spiciness delivers spicy in a different way.)* We could also add garlic for warmth and aromatic quality. And, we can add a touch of sugar for a more balanced tangy flavor.

Most people don't notice secondary flavors because in most dishes they blend in with the other ingredients to fill the whole of flavor perception becoming complimentary flavors.

Some more examples of secondary flavors would be salty and sweet candy (*juxtaposed sweet*), sweet and sour sauce (*tangy*), pickle brine before it has had anything but salt and vinegar added (*amplified sour*), and soy sauce (*amplified savory*).

To help make it easier for you to understand, here is a breakdown of secondary flavors.

Secondary Flavor Senses Chart

Combined Flavors	Resulting Secondary Flavor
salty + savory	amplified savory
sweet + sour	tangy
salty + sour	amplified sour
salty + sweet	juxtaposed sweet
spicy + sweet	heated sweet

Complimentary and Contradictory Flavors

Flavor works a lot like colors on a color wheel. Some flavors are bright and bold. Some flavors are muted and subtle. But, each flavor works together with the other flavors and senses to build a color of each food. Just as an artist picks colors to paint on canvas, we will pick flavors to paint onto our foods.

Complimentary flavors are flavors that blend together so well that they blend into one single continuous flavor, like amplified savory. Contradictory flavors are flavors that seem like they shouldn't go together, but for some reason they bring out new aspects of each flavor like tangy or juxtaposed sweet.

For a moment, let's pretend we've mixed all of the colors together in a bucket. Depending on the amount of black in the paint, you'll usually end up with some form of brown. What we are trying to do is to blend all the colors, or in this case flavors, until we get some kind of brown. Now, each dish should be its own form of brown and should exemplify the main ingredients.

For example, beef stew should be more savory. Red curries should be spicy and fragrant. Desserts should be sweet. And potato chips [*crisps*] should be salty. This isn't a fact that will change with anything you cook. Just to clarify, when I say we are trying to achieve a "brown," I do not mean that every food should literally be the color brown. What I intend to express is that the flavors of each dish should be well mixed together.

As you can see, understanding flavor is not difficult. But, it is fairly complicated. Always remember, when you are cooking, to take all of your senses into account, not just your sense of taste. When *Cooking for Chemo*, because the senses are out of alignment, it is important to consider which of the fundamental flavors are askew. If salty is overly sensitive, it will make every other flavor fall out of alignment, including the above secondary flavor senses. So, I advise you to always think out the problem to find its root cause. In the case of over sensitivity to salty, reduce the amount of salt in your cooking automatically. In the upcoming lesson, I am going to take these basic concepts and elaborate on them more.

Food For Thought
Think about what you just learned and how it applies to your situation. Ask yourself these questions.

1. What dishes emphasize a singular flavor that you like best?

2. When you create sauces, are you trying to balance flavors, blend flavors, or emphasize certain flavors?

3. What flavor senses are overly sensitive for you right now?

LESSON 4:
HERBS & SPICES
THE NOSE OF YOUR FOOD

Now that we are familiar with taste, its complexities, and the basics of our other senses, we need to talk a little more in depth about smell. Or, what I call "the nose of your food." You can make many fantastic dishes with very basic ingredients like kosher salt, MSG, black pepper, red wine vinegar, and granulated sugar. But, what we want to do is give our food some character and maybe add a few aromatic qualities to give our food even more appeal. To do this, we are going to add spices and herbs. Many times people get confused as to what the differences are between the two. It's very simple.

Spices tend to be derived from the roots, bark, flowers, or seeds of a flavorful plant.

Herbs are dried or fresh leaves of edible plants that impart an aromatic flavor.

To make it easier:

Spices:
cinnamon *(bark)*
nutmeg *(seed)*
cloves *(flower)*
coriander *(seeds)*
cumin *(seed)*
ginger *(root)*
black pepper *(seed)*

Herbs:
oregano *(leaves)*
basil *(leaves)*
thyme *(leaves)*
marjoram *(leaves)*
lavender *(needles)*
rosemary *(needles)*
cilantro *(leafy vegetation of the coriander plant)*

For your convenience, there is a *Herbs and Spices Chart* on **page 318**.

As you'll learn in your cooking journey, eastern cooking styles favor spices and western styles favor herbs. This simply has to do with the local availability of products as the different cultures and cooking techniques developed.

A fantastic way to remember the difference between herbs and spices is:
"Roses are red. Violets are blue. Herbs are green and freshest too!"

I want to take some time to talk about the age of herbs and spices and how it effects the potency of its flavor. Time changes the flavor of everything regardless of whether it is fresh fruit, a fresh steak, or dried foods such as dried spices.

With dried herbs and spices, it is really important that:
1. They stay dry.
2. They are not too old, because they will loose their potency.

Just because something is dried or preserved does not mean that it will keep its strength when it comes to flavor. Simply remember to keep in mind that time can not only diminish the flavor but also alter or change the flavor of your foods. Think about yogurt. Yogurt starts as milk. Then bacterial cultures are added. Time passes and changes the flavor, structure, and consistency of the product resulting in something completely different in the end.

Potency of spices is very important to take into consideration, because measurements used will vary based on the strength of the spice. Oregano that is five years old is not going to be nearly as strong as oregano that was just recently dried. You will have to use a lot more of the five-year-old oregano to compensate for the loss of flavor. Also, certain spices and herbs will actually change flavor and smell over time. This is especially true for herbs like thyme and sage. They get musty and stinky. Cinnamon is an example of a spice that will lose its potency too. You need to know this because recipes will call for a certain amount of an ingredient. And if your seasonings are stale, the recipe will not turn out right. The flavor profile will end up being completely off.

When *Cooking for Chemo*, the strength of a spice is extremely important to take into consideration because of the side effect: nausea. Some spices can induce nausea in certain people and different spices can induce nausea in other people. Cumin is an example of a spice that quite often, but not always, induces nausea. Remember in the very beginning of this book, I told you everyone is different? This is a perfect example of that.

Many times you will blend both herbs and spices to bring out the flavor of whatever food you are preparing. A great rule of thumb is to remember not to over-season, but to start out by under-seasoning. We always want to under-season our food while cooking. We do this because you can always add more seasonings, but not necessarily take away. So when you are seasoning a dish, season with about half the amount of seasoning that the recipe calls for. As the dish gets closer to finishing, taste the dish. Then, using the Roundness of Flavor technique, slowly add the additional seasonings that the recipe will require. Make certain that you are adding these ingredients in small increments. If you follow this method, you will never end up with a meal that is over-seasoned.

This is also important to remember when *Cooking for Chemo*, because sensitivity to different seasonings, herbs, and spices can change as medication concentrations and side effects change. Go slow in your seasoning and have the cancer patient try the recipe as you season it. You are not cooking for your preferences, but the cancer patient's preferences.

You should also keep in mind that you may become more or less sensitive to different seasonings in different recipes depending on the ingredients in the recipe. This is especially true with spicy. Because spicy flavors can vary in strength from brand to brand and even within the product itself, always add just a little bit of spicy at a time. A great example of this is a container of red pepper that I have. One dash of this red pepper is equivalent to 4 or 5 dashes from other bottles from the same manufacturer. This same fact is true for everything that we eat. This is because no two of the same item are identical. Two plum tomatoes, even from the same plant, will not be identical in every way. The same is true for humans, dogs, cats, cabbages, and everything else that is or was ever living. This is simply the nature of life in the universe. Because it was living and growing, it is therefore always unique.

The other thing you need to remember when cooking is that you are not trying to change the flavor of the ingredients, but compliment what you are already cooking. The goal is to bring out the naturally occurring flavors of the ingredients. This is one of the areas of cooking where Chinese and Italian cooking styles agree: always season to emphasize and celebrate how delicious your ingredients are! A good rule of thumb is if both the Chinese and the Italians are doing it, it must be good!

Let's look at an example of seasonings in practice and what they are being used for.

Roasted Chicken with Bouquet Garni

Ingredients
1 family-sized roasting chicken, defrosted

Aromatics
garlic, minced
3 bay leaves
1 sprig rosemary
2 sprigs thyme
1 sprig parsley

Flavor Balancers
kosher salt *(or any course salt)*
black pepper, fine ground
1 tbsp. butter

Recipe Directions
Place the chicken in a roasting pan. Fill the bottom of the pan with 1 inch of water. Melt the butter and apply to the outside of the chicken's skin. Generously apply salt, pepper, and garlic to the outside of the chicken. To make your bouquet garni, tie the following herbs together with cooking twine to make a bundle: 1 sprig rosemary, 2 sprigs thyme, 1 sprig parsley, and 3 bay leaves. Place the bouquet garni in the water. Cover chicken with aluminum foil making certain to keep the edges tight around the roasting pan. Roast at 350° F until breast meat reaches an internal temperature of 165° F *(about two to three hours)*. Baste chicken frequently during cooking to make sure all the flavors get mixed thoroughly.

Chef Tips
Remove aluminum tenting during the last 30 minutes of cooking to give the chicken a nice crispy skin. The broth that the chicken sits in can also be used as gravy or can be filled with veggies before cooking to help soak up all the extra flavor! You can also alternatively place the bouquet garni in the open cavity of the chicken or chop up the herbs and place them on top of the chicken before baking avoiding having the make a bouquet garni at all.

Dissecting The Recipe

In this recipe, we have the following seasonings to consider: rosemary, thyme, parsley, bay leaves, salt, and black pepper. For ease of discussion, we won't consider garlic a seasoning. We will consider it an aromatic ingredient.

Salt serves several functions in this dish:
1. to help tenderize the meat
2. to bond with the glutamate and nucleotides in the meat, creating a more savory flavor
3. to add saltiness to the dish, helping to establish our Roundness of Flavor
4. acting as a flavor amplifier to the rest of the dish

Black pepper acts as an aromatic agent as well as lighting up those spicy receptors!

Rosemary gives the chicken an aromatic and fragrant richness, emboldening the flavors.

Thyme acts as a lighter version of rosemary adding fragrance to the dish.

Parsley helps to lighten the flavor of the dish by adding freshness.

Bay leaves add aromatic richness as well as increasing the savory flavor of the chicken.

So what we end up with is a rich, savory, and fragrant chicken! These flavors, or tastes, are the basic fundamentals of flavor. They are the beginning of the road to not only cooking, but cooking like a great chef!

Food For Thought
Think about what you just learned and how it applies to your situation. Ask yourself these questions.

1. Do you have any expired herbs or spices in your spice cabinet? If so, pitch them.

2. When seasoning, do you use a minimal amount of seasoning and taste as you go? Or, do you throw all the seasonings in at once and hope for the best?

3. Did you realize the function of aromatic seasonings and ingredients in cooking?

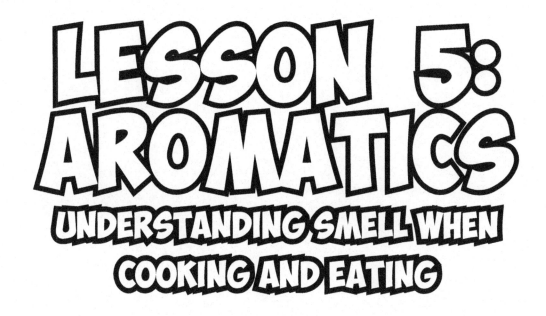

LESSON 5: AROMATICS

UNDERSTANDING SMELL WHEN COOKING AND EATING

Something like 90 percent of all experiences that you have with food are actually nasal related. This is super important to know, because embracing the role that your nose plays in the eating experience will enable you to create richer, fuller eating experiences. This will also help you to understand that appetites are built or destroyed by your nose. I have pointed out earlier in this book that it is the smell of a shepherd's pie that causes you to salivate. So, we will continue with this idea and venture further in-depth into the world of how to use aromatics and your sense of smell to your advantage.

Aromatics

Aromatics, as I had shown previously in this book, include but are not limited to herbs and spices. Each individual food item has a smell all to its own as well. Think of the smell of a grilled steak, oranges, or fresh fish. Each food item has a scent all to its own. We must take this smell into account whenever we are preparing a dish. Remember, our objective in preparing this food is not to change the natural flavors of the food. It is to bring out more natural flavor and emphasize the qualities of our foods.

There is an old saying that goes a bit like this:

"When a guest compliments a French chef, he will reply, 'Thank you very much,' as if it was him and his skill that was being complimented. But an Italian chef will reply, 'Do not thank me. Thank the ingredients.'"

The lesson in this is a truly great chef knows that any dish is made or broken on the constitution of the ingredients that he or she uses. So we must always endeavor to choose quality ingredients and let them tell us how best to serve them. With this in mind, we want to always smell our ingredients every time. An example of this would be if we have a piece of fish. We want to smell it every single time. Fish should never smell fishy, ever. The smell of fishiness is actually a byproduct of decay of the fish proteins. Fish should always smell like the ocean. If it does not smell fresh and clean like the ocean, you should never ever eat it.

This same thought process should be applied to all foods. When you have produce, smell it. What does it smell like? Does your broccoli smell like broccoli? Does your cauliflower smell like cauliflower? Your nose is the fastest indicator that something is amiss. If you open a loaf of bread and it magically smells like cheese, maybe, just maybe you shouldn't be eating that bread. Have you ever smelled sour milk? The first way to tell that milk is bad is simply by giving it a big sniff.

Your sense of smell is actually your strongest sense. You are able to identify a trillion of independent odors. Whereas your eyes can only perceive about 10 million colors. When most people think of smell, they think of dogs. Dogs are always sniffing everything. This is for a very good reason. Through smell, they are able to detect a great many things: food, water, mates, danger, bombs, and even some forms of cancer.

While dogs embrace smell, humans tend to actively shun their sense of smell. People go so far as to look at other people suspiciously when someone smells something. Yes, I know this from personal experience. Don't judge me. There is actually some strong evidence that suggests humans actually put off various odors based on their emotional states. Have you ever heard of someone "stinking of desperation?" As a chef, my sense of smell is my greatest strength. Being able to identify different scents and match them to other complimentary scents is one of the aspects that allows you to become a great chef.

So, why do dogs have it all figured out and humans stick their nose up at the idea of smell? Well, that probably has a bit to do with the desire to feel "civilized" and detached from our primal nature. But that is neither here nor there. What I am going to do is teach you how to regain control of that ever so powerful sense.

The power of your nose can never be understated. It helps you find food. It tells you when to be hungry. It's a defense mechanism. And it protects you from potential harm.

Where this ties into cancer is that chemotherapy treatments, as I have stated previously, misalign your memory association of the food or flavor that you experiencing. Because your sense of smell helps to dictate hunger from a distance, it is absolutely essential that we re-learn these smells and how they make the cancer patient FEEL. This next exercise is non-optional and must be done jointly between caregiver and patient.

Before you do anything else, the very first thing I want you to do is start smelling EVERYTHING! I want you to smell herbs, spices, vinegar, meat, shoes, newspapers, books, computers, vegetables, clean laundry, dirty laundry, and anything else you can get your hands on. I assure you that people will eyeball you very suspiciously. I have a habit of smelling everything. I smell my flatware when I'm out to eat. I smell my food when other people have cooked it for me. I smell newspapers. I smell my pants and even my shoes before I put them on.

The reason I do this is to find out more information about the item I am smelling. Smelling flatware at a restaurant tells me a few things. If it smells like chlorine, I know that they use bleach as their sanitizer and that the flatware has recently been washed. If it smells like food, I know that it hasn't been washed and that I should get a different fork.

Smelling food tells me many things about it as well. I can tell the doneness of food by scent. If it is a steak, I can tell if the fat has been cooked long enough to become liquid and move through the meat. I can tell if raw food is past its prime thanks to a signature bacterial odor. I can also tell the pungency and strength of spices so I know how much to use when I am cooking. If I smell my pants, I can tell if they are dirty and if I need to wash them. As you can see, there are a great many uses for smell, both offensive and defensive.

Smelling Game

Let's have fun playing a game! I have filled out a few items for you to practice smelling that you should have around your house! Smell the item in the first box. Then write down *yes or no* in the second box, indicating whether you enjoy the smell or not. In the comments box, make some comments indicating *why you did or didn't* like the smell. After you get done with the pre-written items, continue practicing around your house with foods and seasonings in your home. If you run out of boxes, continue on some loose leaf paper.

Food/Seasoning	Like? Y/N	Comments
cumin		
oregano		
chili powder		
garlic or garlic powder		
mustard		
ketchup		

Let me ask a simple question.

What is the purpose of aromatics in food?

The simple answer is: The aroma or aromatic quality of food in each dish is the defining quality and character that separates it from the other dishes.

Let's use the following foods as an example.

moo shu chicken *(Chinese)*
shredded chicken tacos *(Tex-Mex)*
chicken shawarma sandwich *(Mediterranean-American)*

These 3 meals are all fundamentally very similar. Ultimately, there is a starchy bread-like substance that acts like a wrapper, a crunchy vegetable aspect, and a soft but flavorful protein aspect to each one of these dishes. On paper, these dishes look extremely similar. But as great cooks, we don't care about paper. We care about plates! Plated and placed in front of you, it would be impossible to not tell these dishes apart. This is because each dish uses different herbs, spices, and seasonings.

The shawarma is full of warm cumin and curry flavors.
The shredded chicken tacos have hints of garlic and spiciness.
And the moo shu is both savory and sweet at the same time.

Effectively, three of the same dish done three different ways.

This is why developing our aromatic quality to the dish is so important. We do this by employing herbs and spices into our dishes to give them their distinct flavors.

I have a certain method to my madness when it comes to seasoning. I always season my dishes in a particular order: salty, savory, spicy, sour, and last sweet. But when it comes to adding aromatics, I always add the stronger flavors that need to be extracted throughout the entire dish early in the cooking process. Stronger herbs and spices should always be added first.

A perfect example of this is rosemary. I love rosemary! When I use rosemary in cooking, I always incorporate it early. The reason is that the aromatic quality of the rosemary is actually found in the oil contained within its needles. It is this scented oil that we are trying to incorporate throughout our entire dish. The best way to extract this is to smash the needles with a flat side of a knife and then incorporate it with hot oil. This will allow the oils to migrate out and co-mingle with the rest of the fats in the dish. This allows it to thoroughly coat every surface. We want to do this early when cooking a dish in order to give the rosemary time to not only be extracted, but to mellow within the dish during the cooking process.

On the opposite end, there are herbs like basil. Basil has such a delicate flavor. Basil is such a tricky plant to use. Because if it is not quite right, you will completely loose the flavor from the basil leaves. In juxtaposition from the rosemary, if you add basil at any time but during the last few moments of cooking, the basil with become ethereal and disappear. Basil is a plant that should never be used as a dried herb. The essence of its flavor is best captured by using thinly sliced fresh leaves. It would preferably be added raw and not cooked. Think of a caprese salad. The raw basil leaves give such a pop of flavor and acts as a palate cleanser. This becomes the quintessential highlight of the dish. It pulls all the flavors together as if by magic.

Whenever we season with our aromatics, we want to first think:

1. When should I add this?
2. And how am I going to get the best flavor out of this ingredient?

Add early: rosemary, cinnamon, cloves, nutmeg, peppers, and oregano.

Add in the middle: thyme, ginger, marjoram, cumin, and turmeric. These flavors don't really take time to develop and can therefore be added at anytime.

Add last: basil, cilantro, parsley, orange blossoms, rose hips, and other lightly flavored seasonings.

For your convenience, I have made a chart of commonly used herbs and spices, their flavors, functions, when they should be added to a dish, and what they are most commonly used with. This chart is found on **page 318**.

Food For Thought
Think about what you just learned and how it applies to your situation. Ask yourself these questions.

1. What smells entice you to eat?

2 What smells ruin your appetite?

LESSON 6:
LEARN YOUR OWN PALATE

Up until now, we have been discussing what flavor is and where it comes from. Understanding the simple culinary theories on flavor is very important. By understanding flavor and its root, you can begin to understand how to develop flavors you love and learn to omit, augment, or modify flavors that you don't like. Many dishes or recipes may also contain a food that you may not care for, but was important for a specific flavor quality that needed to be extracted.

A perfect example of this is in the manufacture of perfume. The best perfumes in the world are not simply sweet or floral. They always have a touch of a bitter or offensive odor that adds complexity to the perfume. The same is true for food as well. Take cumin for example. Quite frankly, raw ground cumin smells like unwashed arm pits. But, when employed with chicken or pork, it becomes a warm and filling spice that grants depth of character.

Before we can begin to build that depth of character, YOU MUST learn through experience the flavors you enjoy and the flavors you dislike. Then you can decide if it is because it is the root flavor, a combination of flavors, or its aromatic quality. In this section, I will be teaching you a proper method for self discovery and how to understand flavor in the real world.

This understanding is extremely important for cancer patients and their caregivers as it enables you to make more informed decisions when cooking and eating. I worked with a woman at one of my speaking engagements who was having difficulty finding foods that she could eat. At this class, I had prepared a large pot of chili for an after class snack. She was eating the crackers with no issues, but was having difficulty eating the chili itself. So as I worked with her, we began isolating the individual senses that were involved in the eating experience to determine WHERE the offensive flavor was coming from. Was it the beans? Was it the cumin? Was it onions? I asked her to pinch her nose and taste the chili. She immediately said that she loved the flavor of it and no longer found it to be offensive. "Ah ha!" I though to myself it must be the smell or aromatic quality of one of the items. Next, we smelled all the individual ingredients and when we got to the cumin she was immediately nauseated. Bing, bang, boom! Right there at that moment we both had an "ah-ha!" moment of understanding that it was the cumin in the dish that she was having trouble with. The conclusion is that by omission of the cumin, she was able to get hungry and eat again with much less difficulty. Start thinking "What foods or seasonings am I having difficulty with?"

Smoking, Drugs, and Prescriptions Affect Your Palate

Right now, I get to be everyone's dad and tell you that you should not smoke. The reason for this is that your ability to perceive and understand flavor is based 100% on your sense of smell, your sense of taste, and your mental sharpness. As you age and develop, not only does your body change, but your palate does as well. Your palate will naturally mature with age, experience, and repeated exposure to new foods and ingredients. Because you learn through experience and develop your palate over time, it can take repeated exposures to a new flavor profile to become familiar with it.

My favorite example is hot and sour soup. This spicy, but sour, Chinese soup is highly offensive to western palates upon your first exposure to it. It is spicy, thin, tangy, and sour. It's a weird combination of flavors. But with repeated exposure, it becomes a delightfully complex and desirable flavor combination. By repeatedly exposing yourself to this soup, you become accustomed to these new and complicated flavors and grow to love them.

When you smoke, it inhibits your ability to taste and smell foods properly. The smoking residue coats both your nose and your tongue. So the first time that you taste Hot and Sour soup, you will experience an incorrect flavor profile, if you are a smoker. Repeated years of smoking actually diminishes your ability to correctly perceive flavors. I strongly urge everyone to quit smoking as soon as possible, because your senses have not been properly exposed to new and complex flavors. This inhibits your ability to grow and develop as a chef. Many people find that once they quit smoking, food and flavors can become completely overwhelming. This is because they have not allowed their palate to grow and evolve over a long period of time. So if you are a smoker, quit smoking today!

The same is true with drugs, chemotherapy, and prescriptions. As each chemical enters your blood stream it changes the way in which you perceive food and flavors. Heck if chemotherapy didn't affect your perceptions, I would have had no reason whatsoever to write this book! Remember to keep in mind that as treatments continue and drug concentrations change in the body the cancer patient's perception of food and flavors will change as well.

How to Pick Out Flavors

Tasting is the very first sense that you need to have mastery over. As I have discussed previously in this book, there are 5 basic flavors that your tongue tastes. They are salty, savory, spicy, sour, and sweet. These basic flavors are the building blocks to create rounded dishes for every situation. So that's all fine in theory, but how does that apply to real world applications?

Just as I have told you to start smelling everything. You need to begin tasting everything. Just like I taught you in our very first exercise, make sure to pinch your nose as you are tasting things so that you are only tasting it and not smelling it. Start with simple seasonings, herbs, spices, and then move on to simple foods that may be eaten by themselves. For example: apples, carrots, and celery. Begin to taste and experiment with the different pieces inside of the food. Did you know that the peel of an apple tastes completely different than the inside? As you begin to taste and experiment with different foods, you will begin to grow and understand your palate even more.

Because each person is unique and completely different than other people, your experience with each food will be unique as well. There is the old saying, "How do I know that the colors you see are the same colors that I see?" While it is more likely that everybody perceives colors the same way, the spirit that you should take away is that your experience will be unique.

What I mean by this is that you may taste more salt or more sweet in a dish than I do. You need to learn to what degree you perceive these flavors. This is so, that as you cook, you will have a reference point to understand whether or not other people will enjoy your cooking as well. This is especially true for cancer patients. We as caregivers need to understand what flavors taste like to them so that as we cook for their preferences we can imagine what it tastes like to the cancer patient.

To this effect, I, for a very long time, was a classic over-seasoner. I guess that I just got so excited about seasoning the food that I would always put too much in the dish, and it would overwhelm everyone that I was cooking for. But by learning that my perception of seasonings was more muted than other people, I was able to tone down the seasonings to a level that was more in line with other peoples' expectations and palates.

How to Pick Out Individual Scents and Smells

Smell is far more complicated than taste. It is composed of a trillion unique scents and odors.

The two things you need to do when smelling an item are:

1. Use association. "What does this smell like to me?" "Is it similar to anything I have had before?"
2. What is the strength of this odor?

Use Association
The human brain, in all of its glorious majesty, works best when ideas can be pigeon-holed. What this means is that people have short attention spans. We will take the shortest bit of information about an idea and stuff it away in our brains. When you smell an item, it is much more productive to build an association than to attempt to understand a new concept. In text, this all seems very confusing, but I have a few examples that will help.

Example 1
Star anise, licorice, worm-wood, basil, and fennel all have similar flavors. The most common association of their flavor is that it tastes similar to licorice. By understanding that all of these flavors are similar, you have now associated these flavors with each other. This becomes extremely helpful when you are cooking with unfamiliar ingredients. I know that fennel, anise, and basil all pair well with pork. I know that licorice and worm-wood pair well with sugar. By using association of these ideas, I may deduce that fennel must go well with sugar and that licorice must go well with pork.

Example 2
Onions, scallions, shallots, garlic, and leeks all have a similar flavor profile. Just like the example above, by understanding that each one of these has a similar flavor, I may find new uses for each ingredient. Liver is most commonly accompanied by onions. But for a change in flavor, why couldn't I pair liver with leeks?

By learning what a flavor reminds you of and is similar to, you may find new and interesting combinations. This also helps with thinking on your feet. What if you are out of an ingredient? By using associations, you can still complete your dish by using similar flavors.

Associations also help when *Cooking for Chemo*, as you can quickly eliminate offensive odors from dishes before they become a problem. If broccoli is too stinky to be palatable, we can deduce that cauliflower will be too stinky as well.

Inversely, associations can help keep you on the right track for flavors that your loved one enjoys. If the cancer patient is enjoying Tex-Mex tacos, its not too much of a stretch to believe that they will enjoy red curry, chili, and other dishes full of cumin.

What is the Strength of This Odor?
The second major defining quality of an odor is in its strength. The proper word for this is the term "pungency." Something that is very pungent has a high strength of odor. Something that has low pungency has a very weak strength of odor. Pungency has absolutely nothing to do with quality or character of a smell. It is neither positive nor negative. Pungency simply defines the quantity of smell.

Example 1
Roses have an extremely weak and delicate scent. When you walk into a room with roses you may not even notice their scent, because other smells can mask the roses very easily. This is because roses have a low pungency.

Example 2
Rotting fish is an extremely pungent smell. The smell of rotting fish will overpower any other local smells. This smell is so pungent that you may not even have to be in the same room (*or same building*) as the rotting fish to know that it is there.

This is extremely important to consider for cancer patients as many cancer patients have difficulty with overly pungent scents. Many times these very strong smells can overpower the cancer patient's appetite. At best, it can diminish the appetite. And at worst, it can induce a full on nausea attack. When *Cooking for Chemo*, unless your loved one is only having success with pungent scents, try to avoid pungent scents.

Examples of pungent foods: broccoli, cauliflower, eggs, kimchi, pickles, canned fish

As I had encouraged you earlier, you really do need to begin to smell everything possible. Your sense of smell is where you create nuanced flavors and find your true mastery of food. Go out and sniff things until your friends and family stare at you like a weirdo. This really is the only way to build your sense of smell database and learn your palate.

How to Deconstruct a Recipe into Its Parts

Being able to deconstruct a recipe will help you adjust your recipes quickly and easily to the cancer patient's preferences. Because you will be able to identify the function of each component in the recipe, you will then be able to make substitutions, adjustments, or create a whole new recipe. This, in essence, is the key to true food mastery. Once you can identify each part that an ingredient plays in a recipe, the sky is the limit! No culinary style or recipe will be daunting or mysterious.

The best way to identify the parts of a recipe is of course by studying recipes and then labeling each component and what their function is. Think of this process like a culinary frog dissection. The good news is there will not be a smelly, stinky frog in front of you unless your recipe is frog legs.

I am now going to teach you how to identify each component and their purpose. Because ingredients often have multiple purposes inside of a dish, we will keep it simple and identify the main purpose of each component.

Recipe Components

Flavor Balancers

These are the ingredients that focus on balancing and manipulating the 5 flavors of salty, savory, spicy, sour, and sweet. These are also the ingredients that influence the perceived weight of a dish in your mouth. These ingredients are the defining qualities inside of Roundness of Flavor and Palate Cleansing. These ingredients may very well possess an aromatic quality, but their primary use in cooking is for balancing the 5 flavors that you perceive with your tongue.

Examples of flavor balancers: kosher salt, MSG, soy sauce, black pepper, cayenne pepper, red wine vinegar, apple cider vinegar, honey, and sugar.

Aromatics -Seasonings and Spices

These are the components that are easiest to identify. These components are your herbs and spices that you will use to define the aromatic quality of the dish. Remember, aromatic quality means everything that you experience with your nose alone.

Examples of aromatics: curry powder, cinnamon, oregano, rosemary, sage, and thyme.

These ingredients focus primarily on the aromatic aspect of the eating experience. We do not use these components for their mouth taste. Even though each of those ingredients has a taste inside of your mouth, we are using these to expressly influence your nose's perception of what you are eating.

Where this can be confusing is with herbs like basil, cilantro, mint and parsley. We use these 4 specific herbs, not for their aromatic quality, but for their ability to affect taste and cleanse your palate while eating. This is the reason that I place these 4 herbs in flavor balancers, not aromatics.

Protein Aspect

Protein really makes what you are eating a meal. Without protein in your dish, it is simply a side. Protein-less dishes are not very filling, nor are they satisfying. One of the reasons that ice cream is so filling is because of the protein found in the milk.

Take a Caesar's salad for example. By itself, it is at very best a side dish. But, add sliced grilled chicken to it and now you have a meal. This is why protein is so important. It completes a dish and gives it a focus.

Examples of animal protein: chicken, turkey, beef, pork, lamb, fish, shellfish, eggs, milk, cheese, and yogurt.

Examples of non-animal protein: tofu, legumes, nuts, beans, and lentils.

Starch/Carbohydrate Aspect

Starches and carbohydrates fill out your meal. They are made out of grain crops which are staples of food across the entirety of the world.

Examples of starches/carbohydrates: potatoes, rice, wheat, cornmeal, bread, barley, granola, and oatmeal.

Vegetable/Fruit Aspect

Vegetables and fruits are what add variety to your dishes. By changing out your vegetables, you can easily change the character of your dish, with the least modification.

Examples of vegetables and fruits: carrots, celery, broccoli, cabbage, mushrooms, onions, cucumbers, olives, bell peppers, squashes, tomatoes, apples, pears, grapes, and bananas.

There are few items that are typically considered vegetables, but are better classified in other categories. A few examples of this are: peas, corn *(maize)* kernels, and green beans.

Peas are legumes not vegetables, so they belong in protein. Corn *(maize)* kernels are actually a grain and belong in carbohydrates. Green beans are unripened bean pods and are actually a protein.

Binders/Thickeners

This is a fairly self explanatory section. These are the ingredients who have the singular function in the dish of binding the ingredients together, tying the ingredients together, or thickening a sauce that the ingredients sit in. This gets a little convoluted because sometimes an ingredient can be a binder and other times it can be something else. This is where your ability to discern the function of the ingredient becomes incredibly important. Remember to think about primary function in a specific recipe, not in all recipes.

Examples of binders/thickeners: wheat flour, rice flour, cornstarch, tapioca flour, potato starch, roux, eggs, and condensed cream soups.

Defining Ingredients

A defining ingredient is a specific ingredient inside of a recipe that could normally be defined in another category. IE: protein, carbohydrate, or vegetable. But inside of one specific recipe, it does not serve any other purpose but to define the character or quality of a dish.

The defining ingredients are never the main aspect of the dish. They are the supporting players who help to create the dish and emphasize the main players.

Take a television show for example. You have the main character who has conflict with his environment or other people. He is surrounded by supporting characters that help to define the role of the main character in the TV show. Let's use the classic sitcom Seinfeld as an example. Jerry is the main character. And the whole show is about him, his life, and his experiences. Let's imagine there is an episode where Jerry simply sits in his living room and stares blankly at the wall for 30 minutes. The main character has not changed. He is still himself, but you know nothing about him because there is nothing for him to interact with or be defined by. If we introduced George, Kramer, or Elaine to this situation, now we have a supporting character with whom Jerry can interact. Let's say for example that George is having trouble at work. He will express these troubles to Jerry. As a result, Jerry will react to George's influence. Through this interaction, Jerry's qualities are defined. This is exactly what a defining ingredient does inside of a recipe.

A defining ingredient interacts with the main ingredient and helps it to define itself within the recipe, making it more interesting. Very specifically, inside of a baked potato soup you have shredded cheddar cheese. While cheese is a protein, you are not using the cheese inside of the dish as a protein. You are using cheddar cheese to define the soup by adding a rich, tangy flavor and enhance the smooth cream sauce that makes up the soup base. This is why it is a defining ingredient and not a protein in this instance. Without the cheddar cheese, the soup would be bland and uninteresting.

So remember, a defining ingredient is never the main character but is always a supporting character that helps to define the main character inside of a dish.

Modifying Ingredients

Modifying ingredients are exactly the opposite of thickeners and binders. They specifically reduce the thickness of a recipe. They are always simple ingredients that change the thickness or increase the liquid content of a recipe. These are always liquid ingredients and are used to counter-act the density of thickeners and binders.

Examples of modifying ingredients: water, wine, milk, cream, vegetable juice, chicken broth, and beef broth.

Identifying What You Like and Don't Like

Once you can break down a recipe into its components, it is much more simple to identify what flavors inside of a dish you find pleasant and those that you find offensive. The hardest part is identifying the function of each component, which we just learned how to do. Identifying what you like and don't like really is as simple as identifying the taste, smell, and texture of each ingredient. Let's break these 3 ideas down and teach you how to identify them.

Taste

Identifying a taste you do not like really is quite simple. Just like we did in our taste test earlier, plug your nose and put the ingredient in your mouth. Then you need to identify which taste senses are activated: salty, savory, spicy, sour, or sweet. It could be as simple as one of these flavors or a complex combination of these flavors. What you are simply attempting to do is identify what it is you do like and what you don't like about the taste of this item. Once you can identify the pros and cons of an ingredient, you may then use the Roundness of Flavor technique to balance out and compensate for the taste of that item. Refer to the adjusting flavor chart on **page 33** for more specific instruction.

Smell

While smell is a much more complicated sense than taste, it too is actually quite simple to identify smells that you love and smells that you hate. Just like with taste, I will invite you to smell all of the ingredients and seasonings inside of the recipe, taking note of what aspects you enjoy and what aspects you do not.

In my experience, I find that those who have difficulty identifying flavors and smells will report that some tastes are too "spicy" for them. For me, this was always very confusing as I had simply thought that they did not enjoy the actual heat found in a dish. But upon further pressing for information, it was revealed that it was actually a specific spice found inside of the dish. This specific example was cumin. Once I understood that the warmth and aroma of the cumin was what this person found offensive, I was able to remove this spice from the dish and create a satisfactory meal that they loved. I did this while not modifying the actual *spicy taste* of the dish.

Because smells are so influential inside of your cooking, many times a less educated person in the realm of food will misreport what they actually find offensive. It is your duty, as a caregiver, to poke, prod, and investigate further, especially with people who don't know a lot about food. Often upon further examination, which I assure you they will put up a fight about, you will be able to identify what smell they do not care for and deduce how to remedy this inside of your recipe. It is extremely helpful to teach this person some basic taste and smell terminology so that they may be better prepared to communicate effectively the next time they find something objectionable.

Texture

Texture is a make or break item for many people. My brother loves the flavor of mushrooms. But, if you put a slice of portabella mushroom on his pizza, he will have a conniption-fit! The reason for this is very simply that the texture, or mouth feel, of mushrooms is extremely unpleasant and off-putting to him. He finds the slimy texture of cooked mushrooms to be simply unbearable. As you can see, it does not matter if the taste and aroma are appetizing. Texture alone can over rule the approval of both with a veto of its own.

Once you understand that it is the texture, not the taste or smell of an item that is off-putting, it is easy to modify the texture into something your loved one will find appealing. In the mushroom example, what I have learned to do, is to finely dice the mushrooms and then sauté them to make a less detectable slimy texture. This process actually worked out for my benefit, because now the mushrooms express a richer flavor than I could extract from them in their larger cut versions. I encourage you to play around with different sizes of cuts and processing methods, if there is a texture that you find offensive.

At Home Activity
Practice Tasting, Describing, and Investigating Various Food Preferences and Flavors

Directions: The next 10 pages of the book are from *Chef Ryan Callahan's Tasting Journal*. You are to fill out these tasting journal pages with every meal that you cook or eat. The purpose is to get you in the habit of dissecting, and understanding the flavors inside of different foods. When you run out of pages in this book, continue your practice in a separate notebook or pick up a copy of *Chef Ryan Callahan's Tasting Journal*. By keeping a log of what your loved one eats and what their preferences are you will be able to identify trends in food and flavors more easily. This can then be shared with your oncologist and dietitian to develop a more effective dietary plan for you.

The following section explains how to use the tasting journal pages.

Recipe Name
Use this area to document the name of your recipe or meal.

Date and Time Eaten
Use this area to document the time and date that you ate this meal.

Recipe Source
Ever forget where you found a recipe? Filling out this section will help you keep track of your favorite recipes.

Rating
Love a recipe? Hate a recipe? Make some notes to remind yourself.

Ingredients and Seasonings
Documenting the ingredients and seasonings used in a recipe will help you understand what foods are common to certain flavors.

Describe the Taste

Describing the taste will get you into the habit of both describing dishes and understanding the roots of common recipes.

What did you Like?

Put what you loved about a recipe here. Ingredients? Seasonings? Flavor? Texture? Color? Smell?

What did you NOT Like?

Put what you disliked about a recipe here. Ingredients? Seasonings? Flavor? Texture? Color? Smell?

What can you add or subtract?

Learning to cook like a great chef involves some thinking about the ingredients and seasonings inside of a dish. This section is to help you identify ingredients that would benefit a dish and serve as a reminder to add more or subtract certain items to improve the dish next time you cook it.

Describe the Texture

Textures are a key component to the eating experience. Different textures cause different emotional responses. How do different textures make you feel?

Describe the Smell

Tell yourself about the smell of a dish. Did you love it? Did you hate it? Identify the smell and document that experience here.

Additional Tasting Notes

This section is a free-for-all. Write down any other information that is important to you. Was it raining when you ate that bagel? Was it sunny outside? Do you want to note that the eggs you ate were well-done instead of runny? Come up with some fun and helpful notes.

Recipe Name	Date and Time Eaten	Rating
Recipe Source		Est. Calories

Ingredients and Seasonings

Describe the Taste?

What did you Like?

What did you NOT Like?

What can you add or subtract?

Describe the Texture	Describe the Smell
Any Complications?	How did this recipe make you feel?

Additional Tasting Notes

Recipe Name	Date and Time Eaten	Rating
Recipe Source		Est. Calories

Ingredients and Seasonings

Describe the Taste?

What did you Like?

What did you NOT Like?

What can you add or subtract?

Describe the Texture	Describe the Smell
Any Complications?	How did this recipe make you feel?

Additional Tasting Notes

Recipe Name	Date and Time Eaten	Rating

Recipe Source	Est. Calories

Ingredients and Seasonings

Describe the Taste?

What did you Like?

What did you NOT Like?

What can you add or subtract?

Describe the Texture	Describe the Smell
Any Complications?	How did this recipe make you feel?

Additional Tasting Notes

Recipe Name	Date and Time Eaten	Rating
Recipe Source		Est. Calories

Ingredients and Seasonings

_____
_____
_____
_____

Describe the Taste?

_____
_____
_____
_____

What did you Like?

_____
_____
_____
_____

What did you NOT Like?

_____
_____
_____
_____

What can you add or subtract?

_____
_____
_____
_____

Describe the Texture	Describe the Smell
Any Complications?	How did this recipe make you feel?

Additional Tasting Notes

_____
_____
_____
_____
_____
_____
_____

Recipe Name	Date and Time Eaten	Rating
Recipe Source		Est. Calories

Ingredients and Seasonings

Describe the Taste?

What did you Like?

What did you NOT Like?

What can you add or subtract?

Describe the Texture	Describe the Smell
Any Complications?	How did this recipe make you feel?

Additional Tasting Notes

Recipe Name	Date and Time Eaten	Rating

Recipe Source	Est. Calories

Ingredients and Seasonings

Describe the Taste?

What did you Like?

What did you NOT Like?

What can you add or subtract?

Describe the Texture	Describe the Smell
Any Complications?	How did this recipe make you feel?

Additional Tasting Notes

Recipe Name	Date and Time Eaten	Rating
Recipe Source		Est. Calories

Ingredients and Seasonings

Describe the Taste?

What did you Like?

What did you NOT Like?

What can you add or subtract?

Describe the Texture	Describe the Smell
Any Complications?	How did this recipe make you feel?

Additional Tasting Notes

Recipe Name	Date and Time Eaten	Rating
Recipe Source		Est. Calories

Ingredients and Seasonings

Describe the Taste?

What did you Like?

What did you NOT Like?

What can you add or subtract?

Describe the Texture	Describe the Smell
Any Complications?	How did this recipe make you feel?

Additional Tasting Notes

Recipe Name	Date and Time Eaten	Rating
Recipe Source		Est. Calories

Ingredients and Seasonings

Describe the Taste?

What did you Like?

What did you NOT Like?

What can you add or subtract?

Describe the Texture	Describe the Smell
Any Complications?	How did this recipe make you feel?

Additional Tasting Notes

Recipe Name	Date and Time Eaten	Rating

Recipe Source	Est. Calories

Ingredients and Seasonings

Describe the Taste?

What did you Like?

What did you NOT Like?

What can you add or subtract?

Describe the Texture	Describe the Smell
Any Complications?	How did this recipe make you feel?

Additional Tasting Notes

PART 2:
APPLICATION OF COOKING FOR CHEMO

LESSON 7: METALLIC TASTES

Now that we have laid the foundation stones of *Cooking for Chemo*, it is time to explore these ideas and apply them to the specific eating related side effects that may occur during chemotherapy and cancer treatments. **If you have just skipped ahead to this section to find solutions, I would like to strongly urge you to begin with Lesson 1 and work forward like a text book so that you can have a thorough understanding of what is occurring during the tasting and eating experience, and WHY these methods and solutions work.** It is the understanding of the flavor experience that allows you to combat most eating related side effects.

In the previous lessons, we have discussed practical information that you need to know to understand the taste and flavor perception changes that are occurring for the cancer patient. Now, we are going to take a more hands on approach. I am going to teach you how to combat the most common eating related side effects from cancer treatment. These lessons all build on each other. So, even if they are not immediately applicable to your situation, please read all of these so that you are fully equipped to handle anything that comes your way. Remember to come back to these lessons and re-read them for better retention.

How To Combat Metallic Taste

There are two very effective techniques that, when used in conjunction with each other, work very well to combat metallic tastes.

1. Roundness of Flavor
2. Palate Cleansing

Roundness of Flavor
Remember in Lesson 2, we learned about the flavors we taste with our tongue? We will use the salty, savory, spicy, sour and sweet seasoning method to combat metallic tastes, and give our food a delicious flavor in the process.

The key to this is to remember the flavor preferences that you learned and identified in Lesson 6, apply these preferences into your Roundness of Flavor. Identify the flavors that the cancer fighter preferred and apply them into your cooking naturally. Did they prefer the dish more savory? Did they prefer a little sweetness? Consider these individual flavors as you are cooking to make better tasting dishes.

Keep a tasting journal and log notes about every single food item that is eaten, how they reacted, what tastes, smells, or textures worked; and what taste, smells, and textures didn't work. This will help you stay ahead of the changing intensity of side effects. This really is crucial. It gives you a road map to work within and help you to visually identify any patterns that are occurring.

By seasoning your dishes according the Roundness of Flavor chart, you give a better tasting product which also helps with loss of appetite and disinterest in food as well. If the dish tastes good, it adds a positive reinforcement to eating and helps retrain your mind that eating is good and not bad. In addition to this, Roundness of Flavor also takes the next concept, Palate Cleansing, and incorporates it into its seasoning method. Remember, sugar follows vinegar.

Palate Cleansing

Palate Cleansing is a simple, but effective technique that you need to know when you are cooking. Palate Cleansing is extremely important to bring balance to dishes that may feel too heavy in your mouth. It is especially useful in taking heavy dishes, like pot roast, and making them more palatable by lightening the perceived weight of the dish in your mouth. Palate Cleansing is where you use acidic sour flavors to create a lightweight feeling in your mouth and on your tongue when you eat food. Palate Cleansing is an easy to apply cooking technique to use on your loved ones with cancer who can only eat a couple spoonfuls of food before becoming exhausted from eating.

In addition to this, the following palate cleansing techniques are also of great help in overcoming the most common side effect of chemotherapy: metallic tastes. By incorporating palate cleansing techniques into your cooking automatically and organically, you will be able to help overcome metallic tastes without giving it a second thought. When the palate cleansing technique is applied correctly, you won't notice it in your food, and will do it automatically in the search for Roundness of Flavor.

3 Ways To Employ Palate Cleansing

1. Vinegar and Sugar Method

Add 1-2 tablespoons *[15-30ml]* of red wine vinegar and 1-2 tablespoons *[15-30ml]* of granulated sugar during the seasoning part of your recipe when cooking. The vinegar lightens the perceived weight of the dish and the sugar masks the flavor of the vinegar. This technique is by far the easiest technique to use while cooking to overcome metallic tastes. A little bit of vinegar goes a long way, and this technique is best used inside of fully cooked one-pot type dishes. Think pot roast, chicken cacciatore, red beans and rice, chicken and dumplings, clam chowder, beef stew, and any recipe with a sauce. This technique works very well inside of sauces. 2 tablespoons of red wine vinegar is enough for a 7 quart *(6 liter)* batch of chicken and dumplings. But each recipe, and patient's preferences vary. Remember everyone is unique! Start with a smaller amount, allow to cook for a few minutes, and then taste. If the dish isn't light enough, add more vinegar and sugar and repeat the tasting process. Remember to add your seasonings slowly to allow them to cook and give their flavors time to bloom.

2. Fresh Herb Method
Top your finished dish with fresh herbs that naturally Palate Cleanse.

These herbs are:
cilantro *(fresh coriander leaves)*
flat-leaf parsley
basil
mint

This technique adds a delightful, fresh flavor pop to any dish. It also helps with metallic tastes. But, I would not advise using uncooked fresh herbs later in chemotherapy treatments as your immune system may not be able to handle the raw yeasts and bacteria that live on uncooked plants. In the case of basil, you can add it to a hot marinara immediately before serving. This will kill any bacteria or yeasts, and will allow that wonderful fresh basil taste to permeate the sauce.

3. Citric Acid Method
Use fresh citrus juices in your cooking or squeeze them over the top of your finished food.

This includes:
oranges
lemons
limes
grapefruit
blood oranges
clementines

You may notice the pattern in palate cleansing is that the addition of acidity helps to cleanse your palate. There are many types of palate cleansers, but ultimately the most effective ones are acidic in nature. Fresh squeezed lime over some delicious chicken or pork tacos not only lightens the dish, but gives it a whole new level of character and deliciousness!

I would like you to notice how Palate Cleansing uses sour flavor to combat the weight of a dish. If you follow the proper seasoning order *(salty, savory, spicy, sour, and sweet)*, you will naturally use palate cleansers in the effort to obtain Roundness of Flavor. This offers the secondary benefit of reducing metallic tastes, which in itself will help with disinterest in food and loss of appetite. This was an idea that we discussed in Lesson 2 when we learned about the 5 flavors.

Here are a few ingredients that you can incorporate into your cooking that really help with palate cleansing.

Palate Cleansing Ingredients Chart

Palate Cleansing Ingredient	How To Use It
red wine vinegar	add in the middle of cooking
lemon juice	add at the end of cooking
lime juice	apply to food before serving
orange juice	add during cooking
basil	add fresh on top of finished meal
parsley (*Italian flat leaf*)	add fresh on top of finished meal
cilantro (*fresh leaves of a coriander plant*)	add fresh on top of finished meal

One last takeaway from this lesson: Sugar always follows vinegar. Always balance your sour flavors with sweet flavors unless you are intentionally making a sour dish. Sweet really does bring balance to the sour flavors and creates a delightful and enticing flavor combination. You may want to consider lemon-lime flavored drinks and snacks to help with metallic tastes on the go.

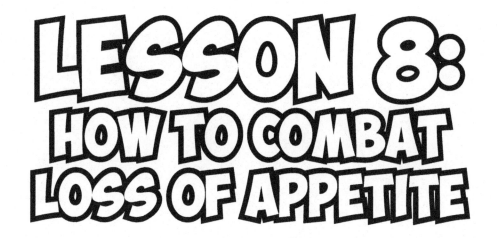

LESSON 8: HOW TO COMBAT LOSS OF APPETITE

Now that we have metallic tastes understood, **I would like to point out that combating metallic tastes has to take into consideration that an appetite is present already.** Metallic tastes are generally found at the finish line of the eating experience. In this lesson, we are going to learn how to build an appetite from a distance so that we can get our loved ones to be hungry and interested in eating all on their own. This is important because appetites are built or diminished from a distance. Metallic tastes only come into the equation once that spoon is inside your loved ones mouth. But, what if your loved one has no interest in food whatsoever? That is the subject of this lesson.

Appetites, very basically, are built on your sense of smell. You do not need to be anywhere close to cooking food to start experiencing it. Your nose is constantly detecting scents and aromas all around you all the time. Think about the smell of a barbeque *(bbq)* restaurant as you drive down the road. A couple sniffs in the proximity of a bbq restaurant and you are suddenly hungry. You do not have to see the bbq, taste the bbq, touch the bbq, or even hear the bbq cooking to know that there is food near by. The same concept is true when we are cooking for cancer patients. These aromas that we smell build or diminish an appetite from a distance.

Learning how to use the power of smell when cooking is probably the single most important part of cooking for any cancer patient going through chemotherapy, followed by the concept of the palate cleanse. When a person eats food, drinks wine, or ingests any kind of substance, the strongest sense associated with this action is not taste, but smell.

When I was learning how to cook, I worked for a chef. Let's call him "Big Chef." Big Chef and I worked at a golf course. We always had trouble getting customers to come eat in the morning. So to get people interested in our food, Big Chef would always have me cook up bacon in the morning. One day, I asked him why we did it. To me, it seemed like a waste to cook all that bacon if no one was going to eat it. What he explained to me was that the smell of the bacon would come out of the kitchen, go into the club house, up through the exhaust vents, and then finally out to the golf course itself. "You see. When people smell bacon, they can't help but get hungry. Somethin' about that bacon that makes people come a runnin'!" What I had yet to realize at the time was that your nose is so powerful it can govern your entire digestive system and ability to reason.

Let's use your dog as an example. If you start cooking bacon, where is your dog going to be? Right there next to you with the biggest set of eyes you've ever seen in your entire life! This is because that sense of smell they possess leads them right to the food every single time. We, as humans, like to feel detached from our animalistic senses. But, the truth of the matter is that regaining control of those senses becomes a very fundamental building block when we cook for cancer patients, especially chemotherapy patients. *Remember your sense of taste only processes 5 flavors, whereas your sense of smell can process over a trillion unique scents.*

Taste is a very basic sense. It only encompasses a few abilities for range and depth. For example: salty, savory, spicy, sour, and sweet. When you experience any other sensation besides these basic flavor and taste perceptions, it is smell or the nose of your food.

The advantage of using smell and targeting your cooking towards the nose is that:

1. It gives you a wider breadth of experience while eating.

2. It allows you to build up the appetite of a cancer patient going through chemotherapy, gently and from a distance, without actually putting food in front of them.

For example, when you have pot roast cooking in the oven, you can smell that the meat is slowly roasting. The fat melting and assimilating into the sauce and the muscle tissue. You can smell all of these things happening through your nose. You can begin to feel hungry without ever seeing the food in person. In dogs, the smell of food can be such a powerful sensation that a dog will salivate without ever seeing the food put in front of them.

How we use the power of smell is by using aromatic herbs and spices *(Lessons 4 and 5)* to trick someone's brain into being hungry. I know that in the case of my mom, I would use slowly sautéing garlic or mushrooms in olive oil or butter to illicit a hunger response.

The other thing we need to keep in mind when using smell is the adverse effect. You will remember this idea from earlier. It is called pungency. *(Lesson 6)*

Think about the most disgusting thing or food you have ever smelled. Maybe it made you feel physically ill. Maybe it was so gross that you actually did vomit? If you didn't have a sense of smell, that would never happen. On this point, we want to think about foods that the person you are cooking for will find smelly, stinky, or pungent and remove them when we are cooking. You will know what these scents are because the two of you will have experimented as I had instructed you in the previous lessons to identify these scents. Remember to write it all down as I had instructed you earlier in this book. This is another place where your tasting journal notes start to come into play.

During chemotherapy, my mom, who would normally be quite happy to scarf down a tuna salad sandwich, became physically ill if I even opened a can in a different room. Think about that. Your sense of smell is so powerful that a person can loose their appetite with out ever actually physically coming in contact with the item that causes the loss of appetite or nausea. She was about 50 feet away, up a flight of stairs, and behind a closed door. This is why being conscious of smells is so important. To drive this point home even further, what you eat and cook for yourself, can have a direct effect on the hunger and ability to eat of a person who is fighting cancer.

Here are some suggestions of food items that may smell delicious and illicit hunger in a cancer patient during chemotherapy. Remember, everyone is different. What builds appetite for one person, may not build an appetite for another. So, keep a tasting journal and experiment.

1. Sautéing any of the following in butter or olive oil:

garlic
onions
mushrooms
green or red peppers

2. Grilling Meats

The smell of grilling meat has a primal effect on the human body. Examples of this would be grilled chicken, seared steak, pan fried bacon.

Think about the kinds of foods that you and your family eat. What are the ones that your family gets excited about? If you can answer this question, you will be on the right path to re-building your loved one's appetite.

The following are food items that I would avoid during chemotherapy. Not because of the nutritional value of these food items, but because of the smell. The smell of these food items may cause you to lose your appetite entirely.

1. canned tuna/canned seafood
2. soft mold ripened cheeses like Brie, Roquefort, Taleggio, etc.
3. preserved and pickled foods like sourbraten, kimchi, pickled eggs, etc.
4. stinky vegetables like cauliflower, cabbage, and broccoli

This by all means is not an all inclusive food list. Each person is different and will have different foods that they love and hate. Like I have said before in this book, each person is unique and as such will have unique reactions to every food. This list is better complied through experimentation than by simply just taking this list as gospel. In your tasting journal, write down and track what smells help make you hungry and what smells make you nauseous.

LESSON 9:
HOW TO UNDERSTAND AND COMBAT NAUSEA

There are many well established ways to combat nausea that range from traditional herbal remedies to modern prescription medications. As I have taught you so far, there are sensory changes that occur during chemotherapy. We need to keep in mind how these changes can cause nausea. Nausea can be the biggest hurdle to combat a loss of appetite. This is because once you have nausea, you will no longer be interested in eating. This results in a missed opportunity for nutrition. Nausea can render the best made dish unappetizing, even if you utilize all of the other cooking techniques inside of this book.

Let's begin by thinking about what can cause nausea. Nausea can be induced by many things, from an imbalance in the inner ear *(think spinning around in circles too fast)* to the smell of something rotten *(hot garbage)*. Nausea can even be induced by the thought of something gross or the sight of something disgusting. Nausea can manifest itself as dizziness or as a full on puke fest. Because this is *Cooking for Chemo*, we are going to focus on the things that we can control and that are mostly food and eating related.

As I have talked about previously in this work, the intensity of a smell is called pungency. In some people, overly pungent smells can cause nausea. In others, they don't bother them at all. This is of course because everyone is different. I see this all the time in my *Cooking for Chemo* classes. We will play the Smell Game, pass around ground cumin and I get to have a good laugh watching everyone's various reactions to the spice. These reactions range from a genuine excitement to a full-on wrinkled "eww" face.

Identifying the Source of Your Nausea

Nausea affects everyone differently. And what makes it so hard to deal with is the fact that often you will not know where the nausea is coming from. Heck, nausea is a side effect of many, if not all, chemotherapy drugs! So let's explore how to identify your source of nausea so that we can treat it and avoid it if possible in the future.

1. Play the smell game to identify potential scents *(spices, herbs, or food)* that are inducing nausea.

Is you nausea induced by a smell like canned tuna? Broccoli? Your spouse's cologne? Take some time to smell the world around you and document it in a notebook so that you can identify potential offending odors and have them removed entirely. The biggest problem with scents inducing nausea is that they do so from a distance. Unlike metallic tastes, which manifest themselves locally, nausea inducing scents can waft in from a distance and completely remove your appetite.

2. Identify whether a pungent scent is what is inducing nausea.

Beyond the actual positive or negative aspects of a scent, are you reacting to the strength of the smell? Cumin is a very pungent, and a quite tasty spice. But if you are sensitive to overly pungent foods or smells, it can induce nausea. Keep track of these pungent scents by writing down how you are reacting to them. Omit or avoid them as necessary.

3. Take the correct strength of your nausea medication.

Your doctor will more than likely prescribe an anti-nausea medication. Don't be brave, just take the medicine. Talk to your doctor about your nausea and more than likely they can prescribe a variety of medications that treat a variety of nausea intensities.

When my mom went through chemotherapy treatments, she had two pills she could take: one for moderate nausea and one emergency pill for severe nausea. In the beginning she only took the moderate nausea pill, which was fine, until she fainted in the bathroom and almost died. I'm not stressing the seriousness of this nearly enough. Nausea can literally kill you. So take the correct medication for your current situation. Work with your oncology team to identify the correct time to take each medication.

4. Dehydration and hunger can cause nausea too.

Drink your fluids! After my mom almost cracked her head open in the bathroom, *(Thank God I was there to catch her!)* we had to rush her to the emergency room where it turned out she was extremely dehydrated. A few bags of water later and she was feeling much better. Dehydration is no joke. It can kill you, and it causes all kinds of crazy side effects from inability to move your muscles to full-on hallucinations. This is the same for hunger as well. Our body tells us when it needs nutrients. We have to eat and drink to stay alive. Because our sense associations are all out of whack, it may be hard to identify that you are hungry and thirsty. I know personally, that being hungry for me used to manifest itself as a shakiness in my hands and arms. Now, it manifests itself as nausea and a headache. Your indicators can change, keep notes and work with your caregiver to identify when you need to eat and drink. My wife knows that I need to eat before I even do.

Combating Nausea Beyond Your Prescriptions

Now that we have been able to identify where the nausea is coming from, here are some ways to avoid or treat nausea that have worked for other people. There are many options for herbal and folk remedies that have been time tested to combat mild nausea. Here are a few of my recommendations that worked for us.

1. Peppermint

It is available in tea and candy form. Peppermint has long been used as a folk remedy for nausea. I can say that it does work for mild to moderate nausea. For us, it seemed to be that the peppermint candies or breath mints worked a little better than the peppermint teas. This is most likely because the intensity of the mint is much higher in breath mints than in tea.

2. Ginger

A classic sore stomach soother. Ginger, which originated in east Asia, has been in use for thousands of years to sooth a sore stomach. It is available as a fresh root, a dried powder, a tea, or in soda form. Ginger does in fact work for mild to moderate nausea. Be warned in advance though, ginger is in fact a warm spicy flavor, not a mild sweet flavor. Its warm spicy flavor often takes people by surprise!

Ginger can be cooked into soups very easily, and its aromatic quality does change the flavor of many dishes. At first this can be distracting, but as you get used to the new flavor you'll grow to love its comforting aroma. If you do decide to work ginger into your recipes, fresh ginger root is the best of all the flavors. Remove the ginger root before serving the dish though, as raw ginger can have an overpowering flavor when chewed.

3. Sipping Liquids

For mild nausea, a warm cup of soup broth to sip can help to set you right. In addition to this, soup broth has a caloric value which can be extremely helpful for those having trouble getting necessary nutrients into their bodies. You can also slowly sip water. This can help with mild nausea. Make certain not to quickly drink the liquids. An upset and sudden influx of fluids can cause the inverse of the intended effect and cause you to become extremely nauseous!

4. Rubbing Alcohol *(isopropyl alcohol)*

This is a technique that a post-surgical nurse taught me. When you are extremely nauseous, take a cap full of rubbing alcohol and smell it. Do NOT snort it! Do NOT drink it! But take a few sniffs of the fumes. It will immediately settle your nausea. This technique does not work for everyone, but for those whom it works, it does work extremely well. I can personally vouch for this technique.

5. Farting and Burping

Yes, you read that correctly! Often nausea can be induced by expanding gas in your torso. There are only two ways to release it and that is farting and burping. Are they rude? Yes. Can it be hilarious? Absolutely. But these are necessary bodily functions, so don't worry about being polite and just let 'em rip. Remember, better out than in!

Techniques to Help Avoid Nausea Entirely

As the old expression says "an ounce of prevention is worth a pound of cure." So, is this still true today? While not all nausea can be avoided, here are a few ideas and techniques that you can try to employ in your every day life.

1. Avoid pungent smells.

Pungency is a concept that has to do with the strength of odors. Whereas smell describes the character of an odor. Pungency has to do with the strength irregardless of the pleasantry. For example, roses have a low pungency and it can be hard to detect their scent. Inversely, rotting fish has a very high pungency. Foods that have high pungency can induce nausea more easily than other foods.

2. Use soothing herbs in your cooking.

Rosemary, sage, thyme, basil, parsley, and ginger all have soothing scents that can help to keep nausea from occurring while eating.

3. Mask pungent smells when necessary.

A great way to mask pungent smells is actually through the palate cleansing technique. Red wine vinegar can actually help to remove the pungent scents that foods like brussels sprouts emit during the cooking process. This can help you to make more nutritious meals while still catering for a loved one's preferences.

Hopefully these tips and techniques will get you started on the right path to not only combating nausea, but avoiding it entirely.

LESSON 10: HOW TO ADJUST YOUR COOKING FOR MOUTH SORES

Mouth sores are an often reported and highly painful side effect of cancer and chemotherapy treatment. Mouth sores can be unavoidable as the chemotherapy treatments begin to break down the softer tissues in your body. However, there are some common sense cooking techniques and tips to take into consideration so that we don't exacerbate mouth sores when eating.

1. Be conscious of heat, both thermal and spicy.

While it may be soothing to your throat to drink a nice hot cup of tea or broth, hot liquids can make mouth sores worse by burning the already irritated skin. This will set the healing process back and make it more difficult for your mouth sores to heal quickly.

I normally strongly espouse the use of spicy flavors in cooking. But when you have mouth sores, you want to be very careful with the amount of spiciness that you ingest during treatment. A touch of spice will naturally warm up a dish. However, if you add too much spicy, the burning sensation that spicy seasonings naturally impart in your food will physically burn the open sores in your mouth. This is not something you want, especially when dealing with all the other numerous treatment side effects that occur. A quick tip to balance spicy flavors while you cook is to utilize vinegar to help cool down the spiciness of a recipe.

This is especially important to remember in kids who are fighting cancer. They usually do not have the same level of pain tolerance that an adult has. Any pain added can be excruciating. A perfect example of this are the ear infections that I used to get as a child. At the time, they seemed like the most painful thing that could ever possibly happen to me. But now, being an adult and having much better control of both my body and perception of pain, I am able to tolerate much more painful things on a daily basis.

Remember to keep in mind that everything that happens to a child, happens in a greater magnitude than to an adult. If mouth sores are aggressive, consider low temperature foods. What I mean by this is foods that can either be eaten at room temperature, refrigerator temperature, or freezer temperature. Because hot foods can agitate mouth sores, this can lead to an extremely painful experience.

2. Be texture conscious with your food.

Dry foods like crackers, cookies, chips, and pretzels may taste delicious. But when you have mouth sores, they can be your worst enemy. The abrasive textures and rough edges of these foods can actually rub your mouth sores raw and make them worse. This can sometimes even lead to inadvertent bleeding!

You want to always ensure that all the foods you are eating are soft in texture while you have mouth sores. And while a nice toasted sub sandwich will sound amazing, the fallout from eating such a rough substance is sure to leave you in a raw situation.

With mouth sores, you really need to stick to soft non-abrasive textures. These don't have to be just soups and stews though. You can absolutely eat foods that are softer in texture like cold sandwiches, meals cooked in a slow cooker, pasta, mashed potatoes, smoothies, and the like.

3. Don't let your mouth become too dry.

Use care when ingesting caffeine, salt, acidic foods and liquids. While a nice cup of tea or your favorite cola drink may sound refreshing, the high acidity and caffeine can actually leave you more dehydrated than when you started. Salt, while it has many re-hydrating properties, can actually dry out your mouth if it is taken in excessive quantities.

Make certain to drink lots of fluids during cancer treatment. Don't make it difficult for your mouth to get hydration. The most logical way to stay hydrated is, of course, by ingestion. If possible, frequently sip water and rinse it around your mouth before swallowing. During my mother's cancer treatments, I would physically hold a cup of water with a straw for her to sip every hour to ensure she stayed properly hydrated.

You can also try an over the counter dry mouth rinse. Many oncologists will recommend a dry mouth rise for those with chronic dry mouth. These can help, but are not an end-all-beat-all solution to ending dry mouth. Many oncologists and cancer fighters report success with dry mouth rinses.

Other cancer fighters have reported success with a salt water rinse. Simply add a tablespoon of salt to 8 ounces of water and stir well. Rinse in your mouth like a mouth wash. Spit out the mixture when done. Do not swallow the salt water. It will make you nauseous.

4. Be conscious of overly acidic ingredients.

Lemon juice and vinegar are powerful palate cleansers, but their high acidity can actually cause a burning sensation in your mouth sores. If you are using either citrus juices or vinegars to combat metallic tastes make certain that you are cooking them into the dish or diluting them in some way before you ingest them.

This is really all there is to mouth sores as far as cooking is concerned. Remember to keep a journal and write down what works for you and what does not work for you.

LESSON 11: INABILITY TO CHEW OR SWALLOW

An inability to chew or swallow usually follows forms of head and neck cancer. The very first cooking question that I was ever asked in regards to cancer was about how to combat this problem. So, I feel it is very appropriate to include this information in my books just in case you find yourself in this situation.

Feeding a person who has difficulty chewing or swallowing may seem like an overwhelming task. But, the great news is we can fix this! The primary problems are usually lack of teeth, change in taste, and lack of saliva. What I would recommend are the following: soups, smoothies, and purees.

Purees

A puree is exactly what it sounds like. It is a fully cooked recipe introduced to a blender and liquefied. The good news is a puree tastes exactly like whatever food you made it out of. So, let's use baked potato soup for an example. You would make the baked potato soup as normal, which would normally be filled with big chunks of potato, bacon, and a hearty cream sauce.

At this point, what you would do is either:
1. Use an immersion blender and puree the food inside of the pot. *(like a marinara)*
2. You remove some of the soup from the pot. Add it to an external blender. Then blend.

Two great things about purees are that:
1. They taste exactly like whatever you made them out of.
2. You can alter the consistency.

If your loved one is getting a bit of dry mouth, we can always add excess liquid to the puree to make it more runny. The excess liquid in the dish will make up for the lack of saliva. The trick to this though is not to loose flavor while you are thinning your meal. You still want it to taste good!

My advice on this would be to use whichever of the following ingredients is most appropriate in order to add liquid and moisten the recipe:

chicken broth
beef broth
vegetable broth
cream or whole milk
and other flavorful fluids that are similar to what you are preparing

Always exchange like for like. IE: milk for cream, chicken broth for water, tomato sauce for tomato juice etc. As long as you follow the Roundness of Flavor techniques that are outlined in this book, you will end up with a flavorful product that is very satisfying.

Another great thing about purees is that they can be served hot or cold. Gazpacho is a perfect example of a cold puree. Purees were actually a very fancy way of preparing soups and side dishes in the early 1900's. The act of pulverizing a food product was thought to make digestion easier since it did not require any chewing, but still maintained all of its nutritional value and fiber. There are tons of classical recipes for purees. You just might have to do some digging to find some recipes that you like.

The big key difference between a puree and baby food is adult flavor. Follow the Roundness of Flavor and Palate Cleansing techniques in this cookbook, and you should have absolutely no trouble with this technique.

LESSON 12:
WHAT GOES IN, MUST COME OUT

Because the opposite of ingestion is waste excretion, let's discuss what happens after you get done eating and digesting. Yes, your assumptions are correct. We are going to talk about the big number 2.

As the old saying goes, "What goes up, must come down." The same is true for eating. "What goes in, must come out." Normally, your body simply takes care of everything automatically. But, if you are going too much or going to little, it becomes quite the problem. I am going to give you some real world advice on these two common problems, address their causes, and offer you some helpful solutions that will hopefully enable you to rectify the situation quickly. I promise I won't fart around about this topic either.

Let's first start with some basic biology. When you eat food or drink liquids, they travel through your mouth and into your stomach. After your stomach, they travel into your intestines. Eventually, all of this ends up at the other side coming out as number 1 or number 2. This is your body's way of eliminating waste and chemicals inside the body that have been converted into useful material for your own body. This is a super important function of your body. And if it doesn't work correctly, it can cause all kinds of other back ups in the system.

What's really interesting about digestion is that it is one of the core functions of your body. And yet, many people will go their entire lives without actually giving it any thought until there is a problem.

What To Do If There's No More 2

Generally speaking, an inability to go is caused by dehydration in the lower intestine. This could also be caused by not eating enough fiber or eating too much processed cheese. Other things that can stop you from going are the anesthesia used in surgery, opiate based narcotics found in pain pills, and many chemotherapy drugs will dry you out as well. An inability to go will cause pain, discomfort, bloating, and very stinky smells emanating from your behind. Two easy ways to start things up:

1. Increasing your fiber intake.

Some examples of this would be fibrous vegetables like carrots, celery, mustard greens, radishes, and so much more. All plant material contains fiber. Fiber, as we call it, is actually cellulose. Cellulose makes up the cell walls of plants. This cellulose is what gives plants their firm texture and hardness. The more cellulose a plant contains, the harder it becomes. This is the reason we can build houses out of wood. Humans cannot properly digest cellulose. As a result, we call it indigestible fiber. This indigestible fiber is what pushes things along and acts like a binder for your food as it moves through your digestive track.

2. Increasing your hydration.

The function of your lower intestine is to extract the water from your foods. If you're missing out on some daily commotion, it's a very good chance *(especially if you are on chemotherapy)* that your lower intestine has sucked all the water out of the food. This makes everything dry and painful. This also causes your waste to get stuck. The best solution I have found personally is good old fashioned, grandma approved, prune juice. I recommend drinking a glass or two. Give it some time to work its magic. Because when it works, IT WORKS! Prune juice is filled with all kinds of b vitamins, potassium, fiber, and a special naturally occurring chemical that will get things moving along fast. After the prune juice works it's magic, I recommend drinking a small glass of it a day to help with hydration and to continue to keep things moving.

What To Do If There's Too Much 2

Inversely, not being able to stop going can be just as bad, if not worse. The big concern with going too much is that it will cause rapid dehydration. This can lead to hospitalization. You simply do not want to get dehydrated. Going too much can be caused by a couple of things such as an inability to process whatever you have eaten. This can also be caused by something as dramatic as food borne illness or as simple as your body being unable to process a food item. This happens a lot to people who eat meats that are too heavy or try to eat uncooked veggies during chemotherapy treatment. I remember my mother really wanted a fresh leafy salad mid-way through chemotherapy. But, her body couldn't handle the natural yeast and bacteria found on the outside of uncooked foods and immediately her body rejected them. Remember that there is no way to "wash" yeasts and bacteria off of foods. They must be cooked to be killed. The result from my mom eating a fresh salad during chemotherapy was the exact problem that we are addressing here. Going too much, can also be caused by cancer treatment drugs or a lack of dietary fiber in your diet. Here are some tips to help things from getting worse:

1. Drink plenty of fluids.

Going too much, can cause rapid dehydration. This is an incredibly serious health problem. Don't just drink water. Water is actually not very effective at re-hydrating. Consider sports drinks, fruit juices, and cups of broth to keep your loved one hydrated. The additional salt found in these 3 items will help maintain the moisture in your body.

2. Increase your fiber.

It may seem like the solution to both of these problems are identical. But, we are using them for different reasons. If you are going too much, increasing your fiber can help push out whatever it is your body is rejecting in the first place. This helps you to "dry up" faster.

3. Try over the counter medications like Imodium A-D.

When my mom had this problem, Imodium really helped. I would recommend it as long as your doctor says that it is OK for you to use.

I never thought I would be talking about the other end of business inside of a cookbook. But with cancer patients, there are unique challenges. This, unfortunately, is one of them. Plus, I guess I am kind of the hero here because I have saved you from going into an online forum and having to ask these questions. Now you have solutions in the privacy and comfort of your own home and have maintained your dignity at the same time.

LESSON 13:
HOW TO COOK FOR SOMEONE GOING THROUGH CANCER TREATMENT

Cancer treatments don't just affect the people going through the treatments. A cancer diagnosis affects the family and friends of the person going through them as well. These friends very often want to step up and help their loved one get through such a hard time in their life. Which is great! Very often, this type of support is received in the form of food donations to their loved one with cancer. And while these food donations are very much needed and incredibly helpful, there are a few things to take into consideration before baking your family member or friend a casserole. I have included this information so that you may share it with friends and family that want to help you, but don't know how. *(And haven't read this book.)* This chapter condenses all of the previously learned information into one helpful guide.

Ask these questions BEFORE you start cooking for your friend or family member.

1. Find out what foods the cancer patient is craving.

Ask, "Are there are any foods or specific flavors that are easier for the cancer fighter to eat or are there any foods that get them really excited about eating?"

Cravings are a great thing! They are your body telling your brain how to vocalize the nutrients that your body is lacking. This expresses itself in many different forms from desiring big juicy cheeseburgers to baked beans to chocolate all the way to pickles. By embracing these cravings and catering to our loved ones preferences, we can help to ensure that they will get the nutrients that they need into them during cancer treatment. Listen to what information the craving is giving you. A craving for a cheeseburger may indicate a need for fats or protein. So for this person if they could handle something heavier I would consider making a shepherd's pie, or if they could only tolerate light flavors I would create a strawberry and banana smoothie with chocolate protein powder and a touch of peanut butter. A craving for a salad can be fiber, vitamins, or minerals. For this person I'd probably cook chicken cacciatore with lots of fully cooked, but fresh veggies! Remember that everybody is different and each craving will be different. Also, keep in mind that you are more likely to eat what you like than eat what you don't like. So use these cravings to get extra food into your loved one while you can.

2. Find out what foods or smells are making the cancer patient nauseous.

Ask, "Are there any smells or specific foods that have been making you nauseous?"

Nothing will turn a person's appetite off faster than foods that smell bad to them. An offensive smelling food will dry up someone's appetite faster than water in the desert. These offensive smells are known as pungent smells. We want to do our best to avoid them. If that is not possible, then we need to mask their smell. Broccoli is a major offender in the war against pungency. It is an incredibly healthy choice. But, often times its incorporation into a dish will make your loved one instantly nauseous from its pungent smell. If pungent smells cannot be completely avoided, they can be tempered with fragrant herbs and spices, as well as incorporating 1 tablespoon of red wine vinegar followed by 1 tablespoon of sugar and cooked into the dish. The vinegar will neutralize the scent and the sugar will cover the taste and smell of the vinegar, but still leave its special effects.

3. Remember to take the weight of the food into consideration.

Ask, "What types of foods have you been having the most success with?"

The reason we ask this is because heavier meats like chuck roast tend to be harder on the stomach than simple carbohydrates like rice. But chuck roast has much more calories and protein per ounce than rice does. Depending on your needs, it may be more beneficial to eat the ounce of chuck roast than an ounce of rice, especially if you are having difficulty eating. You need to know what kind of foods they have been having great success with. Then, you can make an informed decision on what foods to choose to cook for them. Heavier foods tend to lead to nausea where simpler foods do not. Think about when you are sick or have a cold. Soups can be the best tasting thing in the entire world.

4. Make food that is easily re-heated and easy to store.

One of the best things you can do is to bring over pre-cooked and pre-portioned meals that can either be frozen or refrigerated, and reheated quickly in the microwave or oven.

The reason we take this into consideration is that cancer is a time of high stress, high anxiety, and surprisingly tight schedules. Most people would assume that cancer treatment involved a lot of sitting around and recovering. When in fact, it is more likely that you will go to multiple specialists per week and be constantly on the run. Those few times that you do have a break, your body is so exhausted that all you can manage to do is sleep. We want our meals to be easily reheat-able and easily stored so that our loved ones can easily grab small bites of food when they have the energy to eat.

Remember that because many cancer fighters are having difficulty eating, they can only eat small portions. So if possible, make portions no larger than your fist and fill as many reusable containers as needed.

5. Think about texture.

Another great question to ask is about the severity of dry mouth and mouth sores. Ask, "Are there any textures that are hurting your mouth?"

Mouth sores can be extremely painful to the point of where their debilitating effects cannot only break your spirit, but also your ability to get nutritious meals into yourself. If mouth sores are really bad, consider meals that can be eaten at room temperature, like a cold soup. Other things you can do are to make sure you use soft textured food and avoid dishes that are overly spicy.

Armed with this information, you can make better choices and become a more effective contributor when you help your family and friends that are going through cancer treatments. Remember, when we cook for a loved one who is going through cancer treatment, we are NOT cooking for our preferences. We are cooking for THEIR preferences.

LESSON 14: BASIC INGREDIENTS YOU SHOULD ALWAYS HAVE IN YOUR KITCHEN

It's time to start discussing the actual cooking part of the cooking experience. But before we do this, let's make sure that we have the right basic ingredients in our kitchen at all times so that we can guarantee a fun and stress free cooking environment. The following list of ingredients are absolute basic requirements that everybody should carry regardless of culinary preference. You will notice that this list focuses on building Roundness of Flavor, not on building aromatic quality. To build aromatic quality in your dishes, you will have to purchase herbs and spices to fill out your culinary repertoire.

The reason I have selected these basic ingredients is because almost any dish can be made and improved using these ingredients. You can truly develop the 5 flavors of salty, savory, spicy, sour, and sweet using the following ingredients. The final 5 ingredients are absolute must haves that are used in the cooking process. They do not specifically build the 5 flavors, but you can't make a cake without flour. And, you cannot sauté without fat.

Ingredient Name	Flavor	Description
kosher salt or sea salt *(coarse ground)*	salty	A very versatile salt, can be used to season a dish or as a marinade. The flakes are made especially for dissolving quickly and easily.
soy sauce	salty and savory	Fermented sauce made from wheat and soy. Buy a high quality soy sauce, as low quality and store brand soy sauce has an inferior flavor and tends to be bitter. I personally use the brand Kikkoman.
MSG	savory	Perfect savory amendment to any dish. It adds pizzazz to any dish or sauce. I recommend picking up a container or package of it at your local Asian market. It tends to be more reasonably priced. The two most common brands are Accent and Aji-No-Moto.
black pepper *(fine ground)*	spicy	Most common of all peppers. Great in anything. Most commonly used as table pepper.
red pepper	spicy	Available as ground or flakes. A spicy pepper that adds a nice kick to dishes.
cayenne pepper	spicy	Normally sold as ground cayenne pepper. Hot but subtle. *Note: Unlike other flavors that mellow or temper with longer cooking, cayenne pepper is unique in that the longer you cook it, the spicier it becomes.*
red wine vinegar	sour	Great vinegar for most anything. Adds a nice clean taste to dishes.

rice vinegar	sour	Traditionally used in Asian cooking. It is sweeter than its western counterpart.
lemon juice	sour	Acidic juice from lemons. Great on seafood and Mediterranean dishes.
lime juice	sour	Acidic juice from limes. Full of vitamin C. Great for tropical, Caribbean, and Central American dishes.
granulated sugar	sweet	Regular old sugar. Extremely versatile. Can be used for sweetening, baking, mixing into coffee, really whatever you need sugar for!
pure olive oil	N/A	Great healthy oil with a low smoke point. This is good for healthy low temperature sautéing.
vegetable oil	N/A	Usually made from soy beans. It has a high smoke point making it ideal for frying or sautéing.
butter	N/A	You will notice my recipes always call for butter over margarine. Butter is natural, contains calcium, and makes everything taste amazing. If desired, you may substitute margarine for butter in equal amounts.
wheat flour	N/A	Great for baking or thickening sauces.
corn starch	N/A	Perfect for thickening sauces or creating crispy crusts on deep fried items.

So Many Salts, So Little Thyme

I get many questions in my cooking classes about salt. I feel this is a very good opportunity to discuss the many different varieties of salts available for purchase. All salts are identical in chemical composition. All are made from the molecule NaCl or sodium chloride. The difference between salts is not in the production or acquisition method, but in the grinding and packaging method. An interesting fact about NaCl, its molecules form an almost perfect cube when they form into crystals.

Salt forms the first step in the seasoning process. This is because it amplifies all other flavors. Also, salt is one of the only seasonings that can actually be absorbed uniformly throughout a food. Because salt naturally exists in all living organisms, all cells can absorb it and will naturally attempt to distribute it throughout a food. This is a side effect of the osmotic process.

When you rub salt on the outside of a pork loin, it creates an over concentration of salt on the outside of the meat. This high amount of salt will pull the moisture out of the pork loin creating a moisture loss inside the pork loin. Then the pork loin will try to absorb that moisture back into the cells to create an equilibrium. This process will occur back and forth over and over again as the excess salt becomes diluted and equally distributed throughout the pork loin creating an equilibrium. This is why when you rub food with salt and let it sit, the exterior will become moist, then dry, and then moist again.

Salts are divided into 2 major categories:

1. Coarse Ground

Coarse ground salts are ground roughly to create large visible flakes of salt. They are best for cooking with because the large visible flakes help keep you from over-salting. In addition to this, they have a lower weight by volume than fine ground salts.

2. Fine Ground

Fine ground salts are the most common type of salts that you will encounter. They are finely ground to make them quick dissolving and easier to dispense from a shaker. They have a higher weight by volume than course ground salts. This can often lead to accidental over-salting.

Major Types of Salts

Table Salt *(iodized salt)*

This fine ground salt is the most common type of salt. You'll find it in salt shakers in restaurants all around the world. This salt has the added benefit of dietary iodine. It is very easy to over-salt with, making your food exceptionally salty. This is the salt that is called for in baking recipes. If your recipe calls for kosher salt, you can convert it to table salt by removing ⅓ of the amount of kosher salt called for in the recipe.

Kosher Salt

This coarse ground salt is beloved in American restaurant kitchens for its large thin flakes. These large thin flakes help you visually identify the amount of salt that has been applied on the outside of meats. The large flakes also have a large surface area which helps with absorption and even distribution of the salt throughout the food. Because of the large flakes, kosher salt has a roughly 30% lower amount of sodium by volume, making it an excellent choice for those who are salt conscious. That being said, because all salts are made of the same molecules it has an identical amount of sodium by weight.

Sea Salt

Sea salt is chemically exactly the same as kosher salt. It is simply salt that has been harvested from the sea. It is typically sold in large grinder containers that you grind by hand at home. Often in countries outside of the US, this is the type of salt that is commonly sold. You can also find it finely ground as table salt or coarsely ground for seasoning. The applications of sea salt are defined by the type of grind used. A coarsely ground sea salt with large flakes will take longer to dissolve than thin flat flakes like kosher salt or tiny finely ground salts. Often, coarsely ground sea salt will find its way on top of pastries and pretzels.

Seasoned Salt

Seasoned salt is a finely ground salt that has had herbs and spices infused into the salt. This salt is specifically used in the seasoning of meats, especially those to be used in grilling or barbecuing. Because the salts carry the flavors of the herbs and spices, it helps to move those flavors deep into the meat as the salt is absorbed into the meat.

Pink Salts and Other Gimmicky Salts

These salts are often touted for their health benefits. I haven't seen any compelling evidence to show that these salts are any better for you than any other salt. Often inside of the salt crystals, trace elements and minerals can be trapped during the crystal formation process. This is what gives these salts their unique colors. From a culinary perspective, they taste identical to all other salts.

Salt Substitute

Of all of the salts listed, this is the only salt not made of Sodium Chloride. This salt is Potassium Chloride (Kcl). It has a similar flavor to NaCl, but it is not quite the same. And, you will taste a difference. Think of it a bit like artificial sweetener. But if you absolutely cannot have salt for dietary reasons, it will do the trick.

MSG, Miso, Soy, and Umami

These days there is a word that you will hear everywhere, especially if you watch the certain cooking and food focused television networks, or go to a higher end restaurant where the chef is trying to be pretentious. That word is "Umami." It is usually followed by the words "Miso" and "Soy" and the combination of the words looks something like "A delicious Miso-Soy broth to really highlight the Umami flavors of the dish." These words don't mean anything to you. But, what they actually mean is that they have used Miso soup base and soy sauce to build the savory flavor. By using these words, they trick you into thinking and believing that this is some kind of magical Asian fusion that only master chef's can make. But all they have done is add MSG to their food in the longest, least understood, and most impractical way imaginable.

The secret here is that 99% of people who cook professionally do not understand the relationship of the 5 flavors and how they work to build flavor. They simply repeat cooking techniques that they learned at other jobs or techniques that they learned from other chefs. Then, they simply repeat them. This lack of understanding leads to a lot of confusion and misinformation that has been disseminated over the years, whether maliciously or unintentionally. This misunderstanding is very specifically about the concept of savory or as the Japanese call it, Umami.

As we have previously discussed, savory is a basic flavor sense that you experience on your tongue. It is the sense that tells you, "this food is full of nutrition." It is most typically associated with the presence of proteins and amino acids, which is why the easiest example of a savory item is a grilled steak.

When chefs use miso, soy sauce, or MSG, what they are doing is adding that savory flavor without having to add extra ingredients like beef, mushrooms, red wine, seaweed, or tomatoes. The most simplified form of the concept of savory is in a seasoning called MSG. This MSG is one sodium ion attached to a very savory and naturally occurring amino acid called "glutamic acid."

There is a lot of controversy surrounding MSG and whether it is good for you, bad for you, or neutral. I would like to clarify exactly what it is, how it is made, and the honest truth behind it. I would like to state that I personally use MSG and see no problems cooking with it whatsoever.

From the USDA: "...MSG is the sodium salt of glutamic acid. Glutamic acid is an amino acid, one of the building blocks of protein. It is found in virtually all food and, in abundance, in food that is high in protein, including meat, poultry, cheeses, and fish."

What MSG does is provide a chemical called glutamate to your tongue. Glutamate is a naturally occurring organic chemical that tells your brain, "This is savory, rich, and delicious." Glutamate occurs naturally in all foods we eat and cook with, except for ones that are not derived from plants, animals, or fungi.

Examples of foods with highly concentrated deposits of glutamate are:
anchovies, kelp, red wine, green tea, soy sauce, miso paste, fish sauce, worchestershire sauce, meats, poultry, and mushrooms.

MSG was discovered by Japanese researcher Kikunae Ikeda in 1908 by creating a crystalline extract of glutamic acid from seaweed. He discovered this while eating miso soup and wondered why a soup with absolutely no meat in it was so savory. For your reference, miso soup is a vegetarian soup broth made with kelp, which is a type of seaweed, and a fermented soy bean paste called miso. He then experimented with the kelp until he could extract a concentrated and dry version of that savory flavor. Today, we know this extract as MSG.

Sometime in the 1920s, Dr. D.Y. Chow, from the National Dyes Company of Hong Kong, developed the process for extracting MSG from wheat. This is how it is still produced today. *(Reference: The Wok, by Gary Lee, Nitty Gritty Cookbooks)* The main problem with MSG is that people use too much in their cooking, because quite frankly it makes everything instantly delicious!

MSG by itself has very little flavor aside from the instant savory feeling in your mouth. But when MSG is applied with salt, it becomes a flavor explosion! The problem here as you can see, is you end up saturating your food with sodium. Sodium can be disastrous for someone with heart disease or high blood pressure. So when I cook and intend to use MSG in addition to salt, I reduce the amount of salt to allow for the extra sodium contained in the MSG.

If you remember back to what we learned about the five flavors, this makes complete sense. Salty flavors amplify the other flavors, and savory flavors are activated in the presence of salt.

The most ground breaking part of MSG is that you can make entirely meatless broths that taste amazing. IE: hot and sour soup, egg drop soup, miso soup, vegetarian vegetable soup, etc. This is especially helpful for vegetarians and vegans who are having trouble making their food taste great.

MSG is typically marketed as "Essence of Umami," "Umami Extract," "Umami Seasoning," or some variation on the word "Umami." Umami is the Japanese word for savory, or the concept of deliciousness, as the researchers who discovered the sense of savory on your tongue were Japanese. While miso, soy sauce, and MSG are savory in taste and can bolster savory flavors, please remember that savory, aka Umami, is not a food product. It is a basic flavor sense found on your tongue.

MSG = a seasoning ingredient
Umami = the flavor sense on your tongue

If you would like some evidence that the MSG scare is still alive and well in peoples consciousness, simply go to your local grocery store, Asian market, or Asian restaurant. You will readily find packages and signs proudly proclaiming "NO ADDED MSG." They have to say NO "ADDED" MSG because glutamic acid is a naturally occurring substance found in almost all food. I am not trying to convince you to put MSG into all of your food. I am simply suggesting it as a convenient seasoning to make your food taste great.

Now if you are still scared of MSG, you can absolutely go the long way around and add some of the other examples I've listed to make your food more savory. *(anchovies, mushrooms, bay leaves, soy sauce, parmesan cheese, tomatoes, etc.)* But, it will take longer, generally cost more, and will require more product weight to make the same flavor. I can make sauce, gravy, and other dishes incredibly savory, decadent, and delicious without the addition of glutamate extract. I just simply don't want you living in fear of MSG because of ill informed and fear based health food movements that have no idea what they are talking about. I personally think it is preposterous whenever I see the words "miso soy broth" and now you will too. Because what they are really trying to say is "MSG broth."

Trust me on this one. Buy MSG from your local Asian market. It will be much cheaper than any other store. *For more great reading on Mono Sodium Glutamate, I recommend reading "It's the Umami, Stupid. Why the Truth About MSG is So Easy to Swallow" by Natasha Geiling, featured in Smithsonian Magazine's website November 8th, 2013.*

LESSON 15: FOOD SAFETY AND SANITATION

Clean vs. Sanitized

There is an old saying, "Cleanliness is next to godliness." This saying is very true when you are cooking. It is especially true when you are cooking for people undergoing chemotherapy. Their immune systems are suppressed. This makes them more susceptible to sickness from food. So, make certain that you thoroughly sanitize every surface in your kitchen every time you begin cooking, switch tasks, and finish cooking!

Now before I go any further, I must explain to you that there is a difference between something that is clean and something that is sanitized.

The simplest way to explain this is: Clean is an aesthetic quality. Sanitized is the state of absence of microorganisms and other contaminants.

For example, just because something looks clean, does not mean it is sanitized and germ free. Let's say I just cut up uncooked chicken on my counter. Then, I wiped off any juice with a dry towel. The surface now looks clean, but the germs and bacteria from the uncooked chicken are still on the counter even though you can't see them. This is actually one of the easiest ways to get food poisoning.

Another way to think about clean is to think about home design shows on HGTV. They'll describe a brand new modern layout as having clean lines. "Clean" in this context actually refers to the minimalist qualities of that design.

Sanitary, on the other hand, is a scientific state. The ugliest and most complicated item in your home can be made sanitary. What we mean by sanitary is "free of bacteria, viruses, allergens, and dirt."

Now when you sanitize a surface, you are decontaminating it or killing any bacteria or germs that you can or cannot see. You sanitize by using a liquid solution that kills germs and bacteria. Everyone has their own preference. But, the point you need to take away is that it has to be a solution that kills bacteria!

This is how we do it in restaurants. We use a solution that is called sani-water *(sanitized water)* to wipe tables and kitchen surfaces. It is a mixture of bleach and water. It is a measurement of 1 tablespoon of bleach to one gallon of hot water. This will yield the desired 200 ppm solution. Doing something as simple as adding bleach to the water will kill all the bacteria and germs on surfaces. Just like adding chlorine to a pool prevents germs from growing in a public pool. If you want to use the bleach and water method, follow the directions on the bottle to achieve the desired results.

You must always sanitize your kitchen surfaces and wash your hands with soap and water to help prevent cross-contamination. Specifically, you must do this every time you:

1. switch tasks
2. touch raw or uncooked food

Cross-Contamination

Cross-contamination is what happens when you contaminate an item through one of the following conditions:

1. not properly sanitizing a surface
2. accidentally carrying over material from another task or
3. forgetting to wash your hands before beginning your next task

What we mean by switching tasks is if you are cutting onions and switch to potatoes, this would not be switching tasks as they both have the same type of bacteria. But if we switch major tasks, like cutting chicken, and then switching to raw potatoes, we need to sanitize in between. When we prepare items, to keep it as sanitary as possible, we start by preparing items with the lowest temperature required to kill bacteria in it, working up to the highest.

Refer to the ***Properly Preparing, Cooking, and Storing Food Charts*** in the next section for proper cooking temperatures and the proper refrigerator storage method to help avoid contamination.

The three easiest ways to get food poisoning are by:

1. not washing your hands
2. not properly sanitizing surfaces before switching tasks *(cross-contamination)*
3. not cooking or reheating your food to the proper temperature

Also, I hope most of you know this. But, just in case I will remind you. Never, ever, let cooked ready to eat food touch uncooked food. I cannot say this enough. Sanitize your surfaces. Wash your hands. Sanitize your surfaces. Wash your hands. And just to drive the point home one last time to make sure you fully understand the high importance of this lesson, SANITIZE YOUR SURFACES AND WASH YOUR HANDS!

Properly Preparing, Cooking, and Storing Food

There is a proper method and order to preparing food that you intend to use, eat, or cook later. The first thing we want to think about is cross-contamination. As we just learned, cross contamination occurs when bacteria from one food item moves to another. This is especially dangerous when it is bacteria that dies at a higher cooking temperature than what the food will be prepared at.

So with this in mind, we will apply the cross-contamination knowledge to how we prepare food. Whenever you are making a dish, for ease and convenience, it is always best to prepare the items you intend to cook ahead of time. Then, place them in sealed storage containers for later use. If you find you are running out of time to make meals, you can always pre-slice or pre-cut up any vegetables you will need throughout the week and store them in the refrigerator for later use.

We had some days that were busy with treatments and doctor visits. And, we had some days where there would be nothing going on. So, I would keep my refrigerator stocked with ready-to-use food items. Some vegetables can also be frozen very easily. Simply slice them up, put them in freezer safe bags, and freeze them. This is especially helpful if you are not consuming your fresh food products as fast as they are going bad. Feel free to experiment and find veggies that work well for you. If you do freeze them, you do have to cook them. Frozen vegetables loose their structure and become incredibly soft after being frozen. This shouldn't be to much of an issue though. It is generally recommended that people with compromised immune systems only eat fully cooked foods. With all these things in mind, let's talk about the proper order to prepare, or prep, for a meal.

We want to prepare all of our food items in this order:

Food Preparation Chart

Order Of Preparation When Cooking	Item To Be Prepared
first	fruits and vegetables
second	ready to eat items or items that will be eaten raw
third	dairy
fourth	seafood
fifth	red meats and pork
last	poultry

Fruits and Vegetables
The proper way to prepare fruits and vegetables is as follows: You want to first thoroughly wash any contaminates away, like dirt, to ensure that no contaminates are present during ingestion. We do not want to remove the skins of thinly skinned foods. The skins contain lots of vitamins, minerals, and

extra fiber. Slice to desired size. Next, we will place the vegetables in sealed containers for storage.

Ready-To-Eat Foods

Ready-to-eat foods are very simple. But, there are few things you need to make sure you take care of to avoid cross-contamination. First, keep ready-to-eat foods in their own container and away from any raw meats. The next thing we need to think about is reheating temperature. This is incredibly important for ready-to-eat foods. If it's yogurt and it's suppose to be cold, it always needs to be under 40°F. If the ready-to-eat food is supposed to be served hot, it needs to be brought to 145°F before serving. This will kill any bacteria that may have formed in the food since its packaging.

Dairy

Dairy items are usually ready to eat in the condition that they are in. But, we need to make sure that they are always stored at 40°F or lower until it is time to consume them. We also need to be careful because dairy products like yogurt and cheese contain active bacteria cultures. This is what gives them their unique and special flavors. We just need to make sure that this friendly bacteria doesn't turn into harmful bacteria. We do this by properly storing and keeping dairy items separate from other items.

Meat

We want to keep all meat separate from each other, as well as from all of the other food groups. At the very least, they all contain some level of bacteria on their surface. The exceptions to this are ground meats and chicken. Those meats have a uniform bacterial disbursement throughout their structure. The reason for this has to do with the specific nature of the processing of those foods in the United States. I can't speak to how other countries process their meat, but this is something that needs to be taken into consideration.

To prepare meats ahead of time, we can cut, season, or prepare these items up to three days in advance if it is going to sit in the refrigerator at 40°F or lower. Or, it can sit in the freezer for an indefinite amount of time. This is assuming they are packaged properly to prevent freezer burn.

If we do prepare our meats ahead of time, we want to make sure they are in their own containers or storage bags that are properly sealed. If preparing several different meats at once, take care to clean your cutting board, knives, and surfaces in between each task. And, remember to always cut items in the above order to help avoid unnecessary cross-contamination.

Properly Cooking Food

Remember that when you cook meats for cancer patients that are going through treatment, the meat needs to be well-done. This is to make certain that any bacteria are dead as a door nail! Well-done temperatures will vary per meat category. Here is a *Proper Cooking Temperatures Chart* to help you know when your meat is fully cooked.

Proper Cooking Temperatures Chart

Meat Item	Cook To Temperature
chicken, turkey, and poultry	165°F
beef, pork, veal, and lamb	155°F
fish, shrimp, other seafood, and veggies	145°F

You need to hold these temperatures for at least 30 seconds to make sure everything is nice and safe to eat. You can find the temperature of a food item with a handy-dandy kitchen thermometer. If you don't have one, I highly recommend that you purchase one!

The temperatures listed above are the prescribed temperatures as recommended by the USDA. These temperatures are almost always in constant flux by a few degrees. So, double check with the USDA website to make sure that these are still the current correct well-done temperatures.

Raw Vegetables

At this point, I think it would be prudent to discuss raw veggies. There is no effective way to decontaminate raw veggies with any accuracy or effectiveness. This means that just because you wash a grape with water doesn't mean the surface bacteria or wild yeasts have been removed. Even if you wash them in straight vinegar there is no guarantee that the microorganisms have been killed. Much of the produce these days is actually sealed with some form of wax or oil to help keep the produce fresh for a longer period of time. This will actually trap the naturally occurring contaminants and cause them to become stuck to the outside of the fruit rendering the washing process ineffective. Because of this, I would not feed anyone going through cancer treatment raw veggies or raw fruit. Especially, if they have a compromised immune system. This is simply a better safe than sorry path that I take. It only takes a few bacteria getting into your body to give you violent food poisoning. This causes diarrhea, vomiting, and generally making someone who is already fighting cancer have to fight even harder for no reason. Diarrhea and vomiting can cause extreme dehydration. This can cause death in vulnerable populations. Food poisoning is simply not worth the risk. I know that about halfway through chemo, my mom was craving a salad. I eventually caved-in and prepared one for her. Unfortunately, her body simply couldn't process the raw greens. Her body then rejected the salad.

Once I was asked if it was okay to quite literally wash veggies with soap and water, like you would wash your hands. The answer is NO. In this case, instead of bacteria and wild yeasts, we get a new contaminant called the chemical contaminant. Chemical contaminants are caused by the mixing of chemicals *(usually cleaning chemicals)* and your food. Chemical contaminants can literally kill you. So do **NOT** wash your fruits and veggies with soap, bleach, ammonia, carpet cleaner, or anything else that you believe would help clean them. It's just not worth the risk.

There are still many ways to work fruits and veggies into meals. So, don't lose hope that you won't be able to make complete and healthy meals full of vitamins and minerals. If you have trouble getting complete vitamins, minerals, and nutrients into your meals, you can always use supplements. ALWAYS talk to your doctor and dietitian first before making any changes of this kind.

Properly Storing Food

Storage of foods can be just as important as keeping your work space clean. You want to refrigerate everything at a temperature under 40°F. Refrigerate or freeze all fresh foods immediately when you get them home. If you won't use raw meat right away, just freeze it. It is better to loose a little flavor for overall food safety when cooking for people with compromised immune systems.

Make certain that all leftovers are placed in sealed containers and cooled down as fast as possible. Leftovers are usually good to eat for seven days after preparation. If you want to store food for longer than that, just freeze it.

The seven-day rule can be trumped by the "nose test." If it smells stinky and it shouldn't, don't risk it. Just pitch it.

Proper stacking order in your fridge should be just like we are strictly required by law to keep in a restaurant. Here is a chart that will help keep you from accidentally cross contaminating your food.

Proper Storage and Drip Method Chart

Shelf Level	What Goes On Each Shelf
top shelf	ready-to-consume foods: raw fruits, vegetables, or precooked foods
top-middle shelf	dairy products or anything with a live active bacteria culture: yogurt, salami, cheese
bottom-middle in this order	raw seafood, beef, pork, veal, red meats
bottom shelf	raw poultry, chicken

Home refrigerators are actually built backward from how we are legally required to store food in a restaurant. How they can get away with this, I don't know. Home fridges are designed for space not sanitation.

There is a proper method to store your foods in your refrigerator and freezer. It is called the "drip method." For example, if liquid from a slice of carrot drips down into raw chicken, cooking the chicken at the proper temperature of 165°F will kill any bacteria that the carrot could have contributed. The idea is that any leaking fluids or any downward "drip" or cross-contamination would naturally be wiped out by cooking the food to the proper temperature.

For instance, the reason that we cook seafood to 145°F is because the types of bacteria that naturally occur in these organisms die by 145°F. The bacteria that naturally occurs in beef *(E.coli)* is a naturally occurring intestinal bacteria found in cows. E.coli is dead as a door nail by 155°F. So if E.coli ends up in our chicken, and we cook our chicken to 165°F, that E.coli has long since been passed for at least 10°F. If the reverse were to happen and the naturally occurring salmonella in the chicken ends up in our seafood, it is only cooked to 145°F. So, the fish will still be full of live active salmonella. This will result in an incredibly unpleasant bathroom experience.

Remember, vulnerable populations like children and the elderly have weaker immune systems than adults. A disease that wouldn't even cause a 25 year old to have the sniffles can render a child or elderly person completely bed ridden. To drive this point home even further, think about how many children your great grandparents had. It's usually some astronomical number like 13, 14, or 15 kids. But, only 5 of them survived to adulthood. This is because children do not have the resistance or immunity to disease like an adult has. Resistance simply develops over time. The same is true for the senior population. Their natural immunity slowly breaks down over time. This is why avoiding food poisoning is so important. I know it's very scary, but you should have a healthy fear of food poisoning. This is especially true when anyone you love is going through cancer treatments. That being said, don't lose sleep over it. Just take the temperature of all of your foods as you cook them, keep your surfaces sanitized, avoid cross-contamination, and you'll be just fine!

Defrosting Frozen Food

There are two sure-fire ways to defrost foods and not get sick:

1. Place whatever the frozen item is in the fridge two days before use.
2. Defrost in cold, running water.

To use the running water method, place food item in an air-tight bag and place in a bowl. Fill the bowl with cold water. Allow a trickle of cold water to run from the faucet into the bowl continuously. This allows even heat exchange. Also, the fresh water will prevent bacterial build up. I do not recommend this method unless you seal the item in a bag for two reasons:

1. It is very easy to cross-contaminate your food.
2. The water will wash away the natural flavors of the food.

There is another method I use specifically for ground meat and frozen veggies. I place my frozen ground beef in a covered sauté pan. I make sure to cover the beef in water. Then, I place it on high heat and cook the meat while defrosting it. Your meat won't be in the danger zone *(41–144°F)* for long enough to grow any bacteria. It's also much faster than waiting for it to defrost. This is a perfect defrosting method when you need a cooked ground meat as main ingredient like in tacos or spaghetti bolognese.

Why is it important to properly defrost food?
It is important to keep food out of what we call "the danger zone." Cue music here. The danger zone is the temperatures where wild yeasts, bacteria, and microorganisms thrive and can rapidly reproduce. These microorganisms can cause food poisoning and other related illnesses. The specific temperature is 41°–144°F *[5° - 61°C]*. The key to keeping foods out of this temperature is by defrosting, refrigerating, freezing, and cooking your foods quickly and correctly. When you come home with your groceries, put the frozen foods directly into the freezer, and the refrigerated foods straight into the refrigerator. Don't ever leave raw meat out on the counter-top.

As you can see, safety and sanitation while handling food is extremely important. But as long as you follow these basic food safety rules, you should be able to create delicious meals that keep your loved one happy and healthy. For more information on food safety and sanitation, I urge you to visit the USDA.gov website, or the website of your local health department. They usually both have great resources, print-outs, and training programs to help keep your loved ones safe and healthy.

LESSON 16: BASIC NUTRITION

Introduction to Nutrition

Nutrition is a relatively new idea in the medical community. Nutrition is also an incredibly dry and boring subject that even my wife, Jessie, that helps me write all my books and articles, routinely looses her attention span and possibly even consciousnesses while discussing. Because she is my litmus test on what the average person has the attention span to understand and enjoy, I will try my best to keep this section as brief, entertaining, and to the point as possible.

Before we get too much into nutrition, I have to define what a nutritionist and registered dietitian are.

Nutritionist: In the USA, a nutritionist is a person who offers advice to people on nutritional information. This is typically a self-appointed title and their actual experience and knowledge can vary widely. Be warned, there is no standardization to this title and no testing or accreditation associated with it. Many people become nutritionists when they become personal trainers or fitness instructors. This isn't to say that all nutritionists are unqualified or should not be listened to. Many have the best intentions at heart. But, use caution and common sense when speaking to a nutritionist, simply because they are not medical professionals.

Registered Dietitian: A registered dietitian is a medical professional who is very similar to a nutritionist in their function. In some countries, the word nutritionist is interchangeable with dietitian. A registered dietitian *(RD)* is an expert in nutrients, diets, is certified, and often an employee of a hospital. To be a registered dietitian, you have to have a degree in dietetics and pass a licensing exam. Because of this, dietitians will have a specialty just like any other health care professional. The one you will see most often with cancer treatment is an oncological dietitian. You can identify a dietitian because they will often bare the initials RD LD behind their name. Because dietitians go through a fairly standardized training, they will tend to give you similar advice based on your situation. I do recommend working with a dietitian in conjunction with your oncologist. They can help make certain that you are getting all of the necessary nutrients that your body needs to heal quickly and properly.

Nutrition, in addition to being an incredibly boring topic, is also an incredibly personal topic. Because everyone's body is different, everyone will have different successes and failures with different types of foods and food groups. You must treat your diet uniquely and not blindly follow other peoples advice. Especially not internet advice. If you find it on the internet, it probably isn't true. You are your own best advocate. No one dietary regime will work for everyone. I especially urge you to use caution if you are deciding to try a new dietary program during cancer treatment. A drastic change in your diet can come as a shock to your system and can cause you further complications.

Any changes that you do make in your diet should be introduced slowly. So, I guess what I am saying here is don't try to get fancy. Remember that you already have cancer. Our first objective is to get rid of that cancer. Once your cancer has entered remission, that's when we can try to get fancy and switch things around. I also strongly advise you to work with your dietitian and your doctor to come up with a nutritional plan that works best for you.

There is a lot of misinformation when it comes to food and its relationship to cancer. I need to set your expectations correctly. To date, the only proven treatments for cancer, that I am aware of, are chemotherapy, radiation, and immunotherapy. But to set your expectations correctly, you need to know that food, no matter what you eat, will not cure your cancer. It doesn't matter how much raw food you eat, leafy greens, gluten-free, or whole foods. Food simply does not cure cancer. It is not that I wish to take your hope from you. I simply wish to be realistic with you that there is no miracle cure for cancer. If there was, you could patent it and sell it for any price that you wanted and be the richest person on earth. Remember, cancer is not one disease. It is a group of related diseases. This is the reason why treatment for cancer varies based on the disease.

Now that I have set your expectations correctly, I do need to say that nutrition is important. Nutrition is especially important during cancer treatment. What you eat when you are sick determines your ability to rebuild damaged cells. In the case of children, it determines their ability to continue to grow and develop. Kids need healthy protein, vitamins and minerals, carbohydrates, healthy fats, and fiber in their diet so that they can grow big and strong. This is also important so that their body can heal during and after cancer treatment. Cancer treatment can be very hard on your body. So in the rest of this section, I am going to teach you about macronutrients and a simplified nutritional theory that will make getting healthy rounded meals into your loved one a bit easier.

Introduction to Macronutrients

Macronutrients are large categories of nutrients that our bodies need to continue existing. When we make meals, we need to make certain that we get all of these nutrients into our bodies to the best of our abilities. One of the best ways to do this is by planning meals that get a little bit of the food guide pyramid into each meal. If you are not familiar with the food guide pyramid, simply search Google for "food guide pyramid." It is almost always the first result. Because cancer treatment is so hard on the body, you need to make sure that you are getting plenty of protein, vitamins, and minerals.

Now that we are familiar with the food guide pyramid, we are going to simplify the concept and categorize it into three easy to understand categories.

1. Proteins and Fats

I group these into one group because they normally run hand in hand. Look at a piece of beef, the red part is the protein, and the white part is the fat. Protein needs fat to fuel it. It is easier to manage fat intake by choosing good, healthy sources of lean meats. Foods that are higher in protein than other nutritional sources *(like calcium)* are placed into this category as well. This is why I categorize dairy into this category as opposed to giving it its own category.

Lean proteins have a lower fat content in them than other protein sources. That is why they are called lean proteins. It is easy to over cook these lean proteins which will make them dry and difficult to chew. Another reason I recommend lean proteins is simply because fatty meats, while more tender, can be heavier on a cancer fighters stomach. This is especially true if they are going through intensive chemotherapy.

Examples include: beef, chicken, pork, lamb, veal, fish, eggs, beans, legumes, lentils, tofu, chickpeas, milk, cheese, soy milk, meat substitutes, etc.

2. Carbohydrates

Carbohydrates are a simplified group that usually includes starches *(complex carbohydrates)*, sugars *(simple carbohydrates)*, and non-digestible fiber *(super-complicated carbohydrates)*. Any food that provides more carbohydrate value than other nutrients *(enriched wheat flour)* is placed into this group.

Examples include: wheat, barley, pasta, rice, breads, potatoes, cereal, granola, etc.

3. Vitamins and Minerals

Vitamins and minerals are the category for all foods that don't fall into the other two categories. Primarily, I intend it to reference fruits and vegetables. Fruits and vegetables are some of the best sources of essential vitamins and minerals.

Examples include: fruits, vegetables, juices, supplements, etc.

Why do we need these nutrients in our diet?

Proteins and Fats

What we call proteins are actually a group of macronutrients that are made up of amino acids. There are two kinds of amino acids: essential and non-essential. Essential amino acids must be obtained by eating because the human body cannot produce them on its own. Non-essential amino acids can be produced by your body naturally. These amino acids are what give our food a sense of deliciousness *(umami)*, think back to our 5 flavors lesson. Proteins are used for immune function, tissue repair, growth, making hormones, making enzymes, preserving muscle mass, and helps you rebuild your body after damage has been done *(like chemotherapy or surgery)*.

Protein is an area that all vegan and vegetarian diets struggle with. So if your family practices vegan or vegetarianism, you must be extra vigilant when it comes to sourcing proteins. Think beans, rice, nuts, legumes, and lentils. I recommend animal proteins as your source of protein. Animal proteins have the most complete essential amino acids that your body needs to survive. But if you were not raised eating meat or haven't eaten them in a long time, you will have trouble processing animal protein. Your body simply is not used to it. If you do intend on reintroducing animal proteins, do so slowly and with simple animal proteins like white meat chicken, lean pork, or lean seafood.

I also highly recommend combining animal and vegetable protein sources. Examples of this are chicken, beans, and rice; lentils and sausage; fish and rice; chicken and chickpeas; etc. One of my favorite combos is pitas, grilled chicken, basmati rice, red beans, feta cheese, and a Greek yogurt based sauce.

Fats are used for growth and development. Fat makes up cell membranes. Fat provides cushioning for your organs; helps absorb vitamins A, D, E, and K; and is a great source of energy. Fat molecules contain the most energy of any food source. This is because simple carbohydrates are converted by most living organisms into fat for long term storage. In culinary school, there was an old rule that we had drilled into us over and over again. This was that fat is flavor. We now know, as I have proven in this book, that fat actually isn't flavor. The actual contribution that fat makes to a dish is moistness and energy. Fat also contributes to the feeling of weight in your mouth and stomach. This is why you need to be very careful about the protein sources that you choose. You should stick with lean meats instead of fatty meats. I have paired proteins into the same category because fat is naturally found interspersed inside of muscle tissues. It is also found in other sources of proteins such as nuts, dairy, beans, lentils, and legumes.

One last thing we need to talk about is good fats versus bad fats. Saturated fats and trans fats are generally accepted to increase your risk for heart disease and stroke, as well as gain weight. And let's be honest, we all like to look good! Unsaturated fats are the good kind of fats that are easy to digest and provide great sources of energy. Think avocados, olive oil, and vegetable oils. Don't avoid fats entirely. You need the long term energy in your body. Just simply be aware of the types of fat that you are putting into your body.

Carbohydrates

Carbohydrates are the macronutrients that fuel our bodies. They are the most easily and quickly digested form of energy for the human body. They are necessary for function of the central nervous system, kidneys, brain, muscles, and waste elimination. They are mostly found in starchy foods like pasta, rice, barley, oats, wheat, potatoes, and sugar.

The simplest form of a carbohydrate is called glucose. Glucose is the actual chemical that your body burns to fuel itself. When more complicated forms of glucose are introduced, your body will naturally convert them into instant burning fuel or turn them into fats for long term storage.

Glucose is commonly known as sugar. This is why when you consume sugary foods and drinks, you get an instant burst of energy and a hard crash later. We want to use carbohydrates in conjunction with fats to provide a smooth burning energy throughout the whole day.

One of the main advantages to eating healthy carbohydrates is that they often come paired with vitamins and minerals that your body needs every day. This makes eating healthy carbohydrates a well rounded choice.

Vitamins and Minerals

Vitamins and minerals are a category of essential nutrients that our body requires to function. These vitamins and minerals are most easily found in fruits and vegetables. But, vitamins and minerals can also be found in most other foods. Vitamins help with the regulation and execution of bodily functions. Where as, minerals are used typically to execute a function or build a component. Let's use computers and robots as an example. If your body was a robot, the vitamins would be the pieces of computer software that tell your body how to behave. The minerals would be the nuts and bolts that made up the parts of the robot, as well as specify its functions and abilities. Two specific vitamins and minerals in action, are vitamin C and calcium. Calcium is used to build bones. Vitamin C regulates immune function. Vitamins and minerals are actually a complicated enough subject to justify writing a book all on their own. Just remember that they are necessary. When we think about vitamins and minerals in meal planning, we are simply thinking of the fruit and vegetable component to our meals.

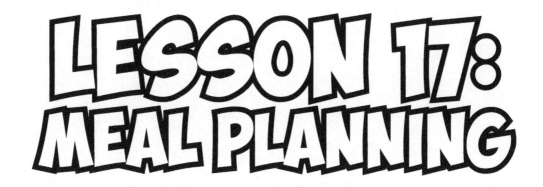

LESSON 17: MEAL PLANNING

Now that we have the boring nuts and bolts of nutrition out of the way. Let's focus on one of my favorite subjects, which is meal planning. Yay! *(Insert jazz hands here.)* Meal planning by definition is exactly what it sounds like. Planning out meals. But where meal planning for me gets really fun, is in the designing of an entire weeks menu.

In this section, I am going to teach you:

1. What are calories?
2. How to make meals that are full of essential nutrients.
3. How to design a menu for the week.

Calories

What are calories? You always hear people talking about calories. Sometimes, they're counting them. Sometimes, they're avoiding them. And other times, they're increasing them. A calorie is not actually something that you can taste, touch, see, or feel. A calorie is not a food item that you eat. It is simply a way of measuring the potential chemical energy contained within a food item. You can use calories to measure the potential energy of pretty much anything including gasoline, kerosene, and anything else combustible. Are you confused yet?

Let me start with the basic scientific definition of a calorie. A calorie is the amount of energy that it takes to raise the temperature of one milliliter of water by one degree Celsius. We use this system of measurement inside of food because when you burn the fats and sugars inside of food, you can actually measure the amount of energy released most easily by using the calorie measurement.

Calories are completely independent from the nutrients that we had spoken about earlier. Calories are not protein, fat, carbohydrates, vitamins, or minerals. When we use calories, we simply use them as a way to measure the amount of potential energy that we are ingesting into our body.

The amount of calories that your body burns can vary wildly. It's determined by a large variety of factors; including how fast your body burns energy naturally, the intensity of physical labor that you do on a daily basis, and a variety of other factors.

To make it simple, there are 3 states that your body exists in:

1. Gaining weight, which is a calorie surplus.
2. Neither gaining nor loosing weight, which is calorie neutral.
3. Loosing weight, which is a calorie deficiency.

Think of your body like a balloon with a slow leak. If we pump more air into the balloon than what escapes through the leak, the balloon will increase in size. If we pump exactly the same amount of air into the balloon as the leak releases, the balloon will maintain the same size. If we pump less air into the balloon than what the leak releases, the balloon will decrease in size. The same is true with human bodies. If you eat too many calories, your body will increase in weight and size. If you eat too few calories, you will loose weight and decrease in size. If you eat just enough calories, you will maintain your weight and size. This is important to know because cancer treatment can cause significant weight gain or significant weight loss.

During cancer treatment, many kids gain weight because of the addition of a drug called Prednisone. Prednisone is a commonly prescribed steroid during cancer treatment. Its most common side effect is to turn cute little children into ravenous beasts who will eat you out of house and home. Because of this hunger, these kids tend to gain a lot of weight during treatment. This is the entire reason we are discussing calories in the first place. It is extremely important to monitor these kids calorie intake so that they do not end up in a state of childhood obesity.

One of the ways that you can combat this ravenous appetite, while reducing calories, is to fill your child's meal with lots of fibrous vegetables. Because fiber cannot be digested, it will sit in your child's stomach, attempting to be processed, and tricking the stomach into thinking it is full for longer. I recommend veggies like carrots and celery. Be warned though there is a very stinky side effect to increasing fiber. I'll let you draw from that what you will.

Another great technique is to increase lean protein while decreasing carbohydrates. When your body is on steroids, it craves protein to build muscle mass. Carbohydrates are full of calories that will not satisfy your child's food lust. So, try working more lean proteins into their meals and see if that helps.

Just to recap. Remember, calories are simply a way of measuring the potential energy inside of food. The amount of calories in each food item is determined by the food itself. We also want to keep track of calories, especially if your child is gaining or loosing weight. Keeping this information in mind will help us as we move through the meal planning section and allow us to make the best decisions for our child. It is also a great idea to record this information as it will help your dietitian with recommendations for your specific situation.

How To Make Meals That Are Full Of Essential Nutrients

The heading to this section could honestly be a book in its own right. In fact, I am pretty sure there are several hundred books available on this topic in any given language. I will try to make this as short and sweet as possible and get straight to the point.

Once you begin cooking at home and taking control of your food, making balanced meals is actually surprisingly simple. You want to make certain that your meals contain all of the nutrients that I had spoken about in the nutrition section. So now, let's talk about the quantities that these nutrients should be prepared in.

Here is my formula for success.

25% of the meal should be proteins and fats and 75% should be carbohydrates, vitamins, and minerals.

The average American household simply eats too much meat. A serving of meat is actually 4 ounces. So, a 16 ounce New York strip steak would actually be 4 servings of meat. If you follow the 25-75 rule, you will end up getting more vegetables and carbohydrates naturally into your meals. This technique also naturally makes well rounded meals without even trying. If you do it right, it will even save you money at the grocery store.

Here's a quick example of what a 25-75 meal would look like:

    4 ounces of grilled chicken breast *(protein)*
    6 ounces of cauliflower and broccoli mix *(vitamins and minerals)*
    6 ounces of basmati rice *(carbohydrates)*

Another example of what a 25-75 meal would look like:

    4 ounces of grilled chicken breast *(protein)*
    4 ounces of sautéed zucchini *(vitamins and minerals)*
    4 ounces of black beans *(carbohydrates)*
    4 ounces of apple slices *(vitamins and minerals)*

In this example, the chicken breast is our source of protein. The zucchini and apples make up two different sources in vitamins and minerals. And, we are using the black beans as our source of carbohydrates. While the black beans would normally be considered a protein, in this example, they are functioning more like a carbohydrate than any other nutrient.

The 25-75 rule is a sliding scale. What that means is that you do not have to have exactly proportional amounts of carbohydrates to vitamins and minerals. You can adjust the proportions based on what you are making and on what works best for your body. If you need to increase the protein, you can always increase the protein. But, you want to make sure that you always keep all

3 of those nutrient categories present at the table for every meal. Remember, you are your own best advocate. The same diet does not work for everyone. You need to learn to listen to your body's cravings and understand what it's telling you. For example, I was the guest on a radio show. A very nice woman called in and felt like she was crazy because during breast cancer treatment she craved trout and baked beans. To her, she felt like she was crazy because most cancer patients can be put off by the smell of fish. But that was her body telling her exactly what she needed. I will explain to you here what I explained to her on the radio show.

Trout is a lean and very easily digestible protein source. Because it is a fish, it is also a great source of omega-3, which is a fatty acid. Baked beans are full of protein, carbohydrates, fat, fiber, and other nutrients that your body needs when it is trying to rebuild cells. Remember, that very often, cancer treatment involves some form of surgery that your body has to heal after. The best nutrient for that job is protein. So do what works best for you and of course work with your dietitians and doctor at the same time.

How To Design A Menu For The Week

Designing a menu is actually really simple once you understand how to do it. Writing a menu is much like creating a successful household budget. You need to take into account every meal and snack that you are going to eat throughout the entire week. The more thorough you are in the designing of the menu, the more successful you will be. To keep this section from getting too long, I am going to teach you the simplified version that I use. This method is the one that I have developed and used. It uses redundant ingredients to help you save money and not waste food. For me, there is no worse feeling than throwing food away that has gone bad from neglect or dis-use.

1. Brainstorm a list of 10 meals that you would like to make for dinner for the week.

10 is not necessarily the rule. What I am trying to convey is that you should brainstorm lots of different ideas so that you can look for opportunities to use common ingredients to help save money and not throw away food. In the beginning, it is a prudent exercise to come up with as many ideas as possible to exercise the newly learned culinary skills that you have acquired from this book. The more you practice, the better and quicker you become at this task.

2. List out underneath each of the meals, the ingredients that it takes to make each of those dishes.

Listing out the ingredients allows you to find the common ingredients and have greater control over your meals. Here, listing out the ingredients also helps you memorize recipes and learn the basic commonalities of different types of dishes.

3. Look for the ingredients that each recipe has in common.

Finding the common ingredients saves you time and money. It allows you to make better decisions before you go to the grocery store.

4. Remove the meals that do not have ingredients in common.

Doing this saves money, time, and your energy. During cancer treatment, using common ingredients makes it easier to prepare your ingredients in advance. This helps make cooking your meals a breeze. For example, if you know that you have 3 recipes that use red onion, you can slice up all the onions you need for the week and place them in a sealed container in the refrigerator to use as you need them. This is a technique that is pulled directly from the restaurant industry. We pre-make, pre-cook, and pre-cut all of the ingredients that go into every appetizer, entrée, or side. We do this because having to cut each ingredient by hand or mix each sauce on the line, as it is ordered, would take too long. Customers would be irate if they had to wait 45 minutes for French toast instead of 10.

5. List out whatever meals you would like for breakfast and their ingredients.

Listing out your meals makes it easier to pick and choose on the fly. Listing out the ingredients for breakfast allows you to find common ingredients from the dinner menu or breakfast menu.

6. If there are ingredients from the dinner menu that can be used for breakfast or lunch, make certain to purchase sufficient quantities.

Not purchasing a sufficient quantity of an ingredient can be frustrating. This can lead to multiple trips to the grocery store, which is a waste of your valuable time. Make certain to account for every instance and every quantity of ingredient that each recipe calls for.

7. Go out and buy all of the ingredients that are on the grocery list.

Buying all of your ingredients at once saves time and money. When you are acting as a caregiver, there are so many activities that take up your time. Something as simple as going to the grocery store can become a massive chore. Save yourself the headache and get it all done the first time around by creating a grocery list.

This is simply the thought process and methodology that I use when preparing a menu for the week.

Give it a try for a few weeks and then you will be able to develop your own techniques that work best for you and your family.

When we are planning our meals, we need to be calorie conscious and to include of all the nutrients that we talked about in the nutrient section. Choose well rounded meals that include all of the nutrient categories. That is where meal planning and nutrition work hand in hand to make you happy and healthier.

Taking control of your food is taking control of your grocery budget. Taking control of your grocery budget allows you take back control a part of your life that cancer will normally send into a tail spin. When you are in control, you are empowered to make better and more effective choices in your life. This leads to a better quality of life overall.

LESSON 18: HOW TO GROCERY SHOP ON A BUDGET

Cancer and chemotherapy treatments are expensive! So when you first start seriously cooking at home, one of the hardest things to avoid is spending too much money on food. Here are a few great tips to help minimize your food expense while maximizing impact.

Tips for Staying on Budget at the Grocery Store

1. Set a realistic monetary food budget and stick to it.

This is probably the hardest aspect of staying on target with your money. But, it's amazing how if you work inside your food budget, how your meals will change in quality and character very quickly. Setting a food budget helps you control your food cost and forces you to learn how much each item costs. This makes it easier to make budget minded decisions while making your menu. The best way to help you stick to your budget is to keep track of how much you are spending while you are shopping. This will help keep you accountable and help you to learn how much your food actually costs.

2. Plan a menu for the week.

When you plan a menu, not only do you have a road map of what you are going to create, but it allows you to cook similarly themed food items. This reduces the need to purchase a lot of unique ingredients. For example, let's say you have a recipe that requires carrots, onions, and celery. This mixture, typically known as mirepoix, forms the backbone of almost every classic western culinary recipe. Just by using the mirepoix mixture, we can make recipes like soup, pot roast, and Shepherd's pie. The variations are endless. Carrots, onions, and celery are budget friendly. They also last a long time in the refrigerator and are full of healthy fiber. So as you can see, using similarly themed ingredients can help you save money on a budget.

3. Don't impulse purchase.

One of the biggest expenses you will run into when buying food at the grocery store is the impulse purchase. I, myself, am extremely guilty of perusing the cheese area and selecting a few things that topple the food budget right over. That's why I always send my wife with the exact list of what I need. She won't come back with extra things like a super rare piece of cheese that I absolutely had to try! Another thing that will make you impulse on food at the grocery store is if you go shopping when you are hungry. Don't buy food when you are hungry. Eat first, then shop!

4. Prep and freeze perishable food items.

Aside from impulse purchasing, food waste is the biggest way to blow your grocery budget! If you are throwing away $20 worth of food every week, that's $20 of loss on your grocery budget. That money could have been better spent in other categories of your life. What we do in our home, is take perishable food items, like fresh veggies, pre-slice them, place them into freezer bags, and simply freeze them for later use. $20 a week adds up to $1040 per year. That can buy a lot of other fun stuff like vacations, movie tickets, and video games. Don't let that much money end up in the trash.

5. Use your leftovers to make other recipes.

A great thing about leftovers is that you can turn them into other recipes. For example, pot roast can be made into beef stew. Roasted chicken breast can be turned into chicken noodle soup. I like to play a game that I call "The Leftovers Game." This is where I try to re-create a recipe of some kind while incorporating leftovers from a completely different recipe. The trick to this is proper seasoning and of course incorporating new and fresh food ingredients as well.

6. Eat your leftovers.

In our house, leftovers translates to one word: lunch. We eat our leftovers for lunch throughout the week. My wife can eat leftovers the next day. I, on the other hand, usually need to wait a few days. Leftovers, if properly stored and sealed, usually stay fresh for about a week in the refrigerator and longer in the freezer.

7. Organic ingredients are expensive.

Organic ingredients are significantly more expensive than their regular everyday counterparts. If you want to eat organic, by all means just go ahead and do it. But, you don't have to feel guilty if you don't. As a caregiver or cancer patient, your drive is to try and eat the most "healthy" foods available. But eating organic food is not in itself a stamp of quality. What makes something "organic" is incredibly misunderstood. What gives you the quality stamp of "caregiver of the year" is by making a conscious effort to make healthier choices in the meals that you are providing your loved one.

Organic ingredients have absolutely no measurable additional nutritional, health, or flavor benefits. An apple, whether organic or conventional, will still have the same nutrients. There are far greater measurable variances based on location grown, type of soil, sun exposure, and many other numerous factors. Because organic ingredients are not treated using modern preservation techniques, they also spoil faster. The best way to get organic food on your table is to grow it yourself. Then, and only then are you getting the freshest ingredients possible on your table.

One of the main reasons that people advocate for the use of organic ingredients is because they claim that organic farmers do not use herbicides or pesticides. That is simply not true. Organic farmers use pesticides on their foods just like conventional farmers do. The only way to guarantee that there are no herbicides or pesticides in your food is to grow your own food and not use herbicides or pesticides.

More on "Going Organic"
Organic ingredients tend to be 3-4 times as expensive as their average everyday counterparts. "Going organic" is not what improves your health or well being. What improves your health or well being is the conscious decision to eat healthier and more complete meals. Adding fruits and veggies to your meals, and omitting pre-packaged and prepared foods will do more for you than switching to organic snack chips.

The best story I've ever heard about the misunderstanding around organic ingredients came from a friend of mine who is a dietitian. She told me about a patient of hers who kept eating cookies when they were not supposed to be. My friend confronted the patient about why they continued to eat so many cookies. The patient justified themselves by explaining that the cookies were organic and therefore healthy for them.

We both laughed for a good long while about that story. But, I am using it today to explain that an organic cookie has the same calories and nutritional benefits of a regular cookie. They are in no way actually different. "Purchasing organic" arose out of a fear of the unknown. The unknown was about herbicides and pesticides being used in the modern production of food. Simply make better and healthier decisions like choosing an orange for a snack instead of a cookie. And, you will be just fine.

For further reading on organic vs. conventional, I am providing the following online sources so that you are completely and totally informed beyond the scope of this work.

Scientific American
http://blogs.scientificamerican.com/science-sushi/httpblogsscientificamericancomscience-sushi20110718mythbusting-101-organic-farming-conventional-agriculture/

Harvard Health Publications
http://www.health.harvard.edu/blog/organic-food-no-more-nutritious-than-conventionally-grown-food-201209055264

Science Direct -Organic food and the impact on human health
http://www.sciencedirect.com/science/article/pii/S1573521411000054

American Journal of Clinical Nutrition -Nutritional quality of organic foods: a systematic review
http://m.ajcn.nutrition.org/content/early/2009/07/29/ajcn.2009.28041.abstract

Medicine Net
http://www.medicinenet.com/script/main/mobileart.asp?articlekey=104207

Mayo Clinic
http://www.mayoclinic.org/healthy-lifestyle/nutrition-and-healthy-eating/in-depth/organic-food/art-20043880?pg=2

Armed with this new knowledge, I am very confident that you will all be able to make better decisions, save money, plan meals, and adjust your calories as appropriate. Remember, cooking is an art that you develop and so are the skills that surround meal planning.

Now, we will move into the recipes section where you can begin to practice everything you just learned.

PART 3: IMPLEMENTATION OF COOKING FOR CHEMO

LESSON 19: PRACTICE RECIPES

Recipes Overview

You made it to the recipes! Yay! Look at how well informed, smarter, and wiser you are now! This is the part where you start to apply what you have just learned. This is the hands-on part where you get to create Roundness of Flavor for your loved one. This is a new way of looking at food and will take some trial and error to learn how to adjust flavor for your loved one going through chemotherapy.

It is not my recipes that are going to help you. It is the culinary theory of how to properly flavor your food that will. So don't skip ahead and start making these recipes without first reading Part 1 and Part 2. You will fail miserably if you cheat and start here. Reference the previous sections as often as needed or until the information I have taught you fully sinks in.

There are 6 categories that this lesson is divided into. In order, the sections are as follows:

1. Main Dishes
2. Side Dishes
3. Snack Recipes
4. Soup Recipes
5. Smoothie Recipes
6. Sauce Recipes

Unlike other cookbooks that have their recipes ordered by time of day or type of food, this book's recipe section is in order of what you will be able to eat at different points during chemotherapy. The recipes are ordered in sections from heaviest in weight to lightest in weight. The reason for this is because at the beginning of chemo you are able to still eat heavy-weighted food items. But as you continue chemotherapy treatments, your stomach and body are only able to handle light-weight food items. This is what happened to by mom. So to make it easier for you, I have ordered the recipes this way. The recipes inside of each section though, are organized in alphabetical order to make it easier to find each recipe.

Remember to use what you have learned. Adjust these recipes for the flavor profile of the chemo patient you are cooking for and allowing for their specific taste changes. So, if that calls for an omission of certain ingredients or seasonings from a recipe and the addition of others, I hereby charge, grant, and empower you with full rights, power, and responsibility to do so.

If and when you do make substitutes, make sure it is an equal substitution, like protein for protein or vegetable for vegetable. Remember you can substitute like for like. For example, if something calls for carrots but you don't like carrots or can no longer eat them, substitute it out for a different kind of vegetable that you can eat, like corn or green beans. In conclusion, don't be afraid to substitute or play around with these recipes as you see fit or require. **Remember, we are cooking for THE CANCER PATIENT'S preferences NOT OUR preferences.**

Please note on these recipes, seasoning amounts are subjective. I have provided what I consider to be a minimum/moderate amount of seasonings available to capture the flavor and essence of the dish. Remember to not over-season and to taste your food as you go. Do not take all recipes as literal truth of measurement, but as an idea of where to start. The purpose of these recipes is to capture the essence of the dish. In doing this, I have provided these general recipe guidelines as minimum estimates of ingredients you should have on-hand to complete the dish. **You do not need to put the full amount of seasonings called for into the recipe, start with half of the called for amount and then add as is necessary.** Again, this is where you apply what you have just learned in this book. **Adjust the seasonings and recipes for the cancer patients flavor preference.**

The amount of seasonings in each recipe are simply how much to allow for, not an exact called for scientific measurement. For example, if you have chicken noodle soup and it calls for a certain amount of egg noodles and you are short that amount, it is not the end of the world. You can still make the recipe by adjusting or compensating for the lack of ingredients. An example on spices, if you are spicy sensitive and the recipe calls for ½ tsp. of cayenne pepper and you know it will be too much, reduce it to ⅛ tsp. or omit all together. Save yourself the trouble of fixing something that never needed to be broken. A specific example of substitutions in my life is when I made chili using chicken breast, pork chops, and baked beans instead of the traditional chili beans and ground beef.

Cooking is a creative art. Don't be afraid to create!

Last, but not least, the recipes are laid out in the following format for educational purposes and for ease of use. I feel that it is extremely important to carry over what I just taught you and lay it out in an easy to use way that helps you practice what you just learned. As all of us caregivers know, time is of the essence. The ability to learn and adapt quickly makes all the difference when trying to feed someone going through chemotherapy.

Name of Recipe

At the top of each page you will see the recipe name. This is what the dish is called.

Recipe Description

This is a description of the dish you are about to make. I did this to help give you a better idea and understanding of the big picture of what you are about to cook. I also used this to throw in some fun facts about different foods and their origins.

Tasting Guidelines

This is probably the single most important section of each recipe. This is the section that helps guide you to what your dish should taste like and how to fix or tilt the dish in the way that enables your loved one to be able to enjoy their food and eat again. Use this to help guide you to get the desired flavor results for your loved one going through chemotherapy.

Ingredients

This is where the ingredients, their amounts, and how they need to be prepared will be listed.

Flavor Balancers

This is where the seasonings *(the 5 flavors)* that are needed for the dish will be listed.

Aromatics

This is where the herbs and spices *(aromatics)* that are not listed in the flavor balancers sections will be. I separated aromatics because I want you to physically see and begin to understand what gives your food its nose and that extra *Umph!*

Recipe Directions

This is how to make the recipe. Remember to fully read through all the information listed for the recipe ahead of time. That will prevent you from making big mistakes when you get to this section and begin making the recipe.

Chef Tips

This is where you find extra information and pro-tips that will help further your knowledge and understanding of why certain things are done the way they are when you are making the recipes.

If you have any questions just email us directly. Also, most basic culinary terminology can be easily found by searching the internet.

With all of that said and done, let's get started!

MAIN DISHES

BEEF STROGANOFF

Recipe Description
A hearty egg noodle and gravy dish. Very easy to prepare and an infinite amount of variations. Odds are you have had this at some point in your life, whether in a school cafeteria, a TV dinner, or a high-end restaurant.

Tasting Guidelines
Taste is rich and savory.
Weight is heavy, but can be balanced with vinegar.
Texture is soft.
Good for people with low to moderate treatment side effects.
Emotional response of a good home cooked meal.
Best categorized as classic Russian.

Ingredients
8-16 oz. beef for stew
¼ c. whole milk
1 package egg noodles, cooked and lightly oiled
1 yellow onion, medium diced
1 small pack portabella mushrooms, chopped
8 oz. sour cream
½ stick butter
1 can cream of mushroom soup
2 packages brown gravy prepared according to mix directions

Flavor Balancers
2 tbsp. dark soy sauce, mushroom flavored
1 tbsp. black pepper
2 tbsp. rice vinegar
1 tbsp. sugar

Aromatics
½ tbsp. rosemary
2 tbsp. Italian flat leaf parsley, chopped

Recipe Directions
Take beef and tenderize with a meat mallet. Place tenderized beef into a mixing bowl, and mix in dark soy sauce until surface is thoroughly coated. Add vinegar and mix thoroughly. Allow to marinate 30 minutes on the counter. In a large sauté pan, melt butter over medium heat. Sweat onion and mushrooms in butter until onions are translucent. Add beef, rosemary, black pepper, and sugar. Cook beef until thoroughly cooked. When beef is thoroughly cooked, stir in brown gravy, cream of mushroom soup, and sour cream, mixing well. Allow to simmer on low heat uncovered for 10 minutes. If sauce is too thick, add milk to thin. Serve over cooked egg noodles. Top with Italian parsley and enjoy.

Chef Tips
This is a really great recipe. It reheats well. If the recipe is a little too heavy, add a little extra red wine vinegar or lemon juice to cut through the weight of the dish.

BROCCOLI CHEESE CASSEROLE (CHICKEN)

Recipe Description

Chicken and broccoli cheese casserole is a classic, go-to dish when you don't have the time to do anything but throw dinner in the oven and hope for the best.

Tasting Guidelines

Taste is cheesy and savory.
Weight is medium, but can be balanced with vinegar and sugar.
Texture is soft.
Good for people with low to moderate side effects.
Emotional response of home cooked love.
Best categorized as a comfort food.

Ingredients

1 lb. chicken breast, cooked and
cut into quarter inch cubes
8 oz. sharp cheddar cheese, shredded
2 c. white rice, cooked
1 package frozen broccoli, chopped
1 small yellow onion, chopped
1 can cream of mushroom
1 can broccoli cheese soup

Flavor Balancers

kosher salt to taste
1 tbsp. soy sauce
black pepper to taste
1 tbsp. red wine vinegar
1 tbsp. sugar

Garnish

fried onions

Recipe Directions

Preheat the oven to 425°F. Combine all ingredients in a large mixing bowl, except for the French onion crisps. After thoroughly mixed, check for consistency. If soup doesn't cover all ingredients thoroughly, add a little bit of milk until mixture is homogeneous. Transfer to a large casserole dish. Pack mixture down into all corners. Cover with French onion crisps and allow to bake uncovered until internal temperature reaches 145°F.

Chef Tips

My mom absolutely loved this dish! And it is super tasty for breakfast, lunch, or dinner. It's full of fat, protein, and carbohydrates, but is also very easy to digest.

This is good for people with mouth sores. It is very soft. If you mix the French onion crisps into the casserole after baked but before serving, they loose their crunchiness but maintain a strong pop of flavor.

A tablespoon of red wine vinegar will lighten the dish. A couple shakes of red pepper will fill out the flavor of the dish. I would highly recommend not adding too much extra sugar as the rice will break down in the casserole naturally imparting sugar. For a more aromatic quality, add some sage and thyme.

CHICKEN, BLACK BEANS, AND RICE

Recipe Description
Black beans and rice is a classic Cuban dish. It is the Caribbean equivalent to New Orleans famous red beans and rice. This dish features a lighter spice palate and a twist of lime, creating a light, refreshing dish that is especially good for those plagued with metallic tastes and mouth sores.

Tasting Guidelines
Taste is light, but filling.
Weight is light, but can be balanced with extra savory.
Texture is soft.
Good for people with low to severe treatment side effects.
Emotional response of light yet refreshing meal.
Best categorized as Caribbean comfort food.

Ingredients
3 chicken breasts, thawed and uncooked
1 box black beans and rice mix

Flavor Balancers
kosher salt to taste
black pepper to taste
1 lime *(for the juice)*

Recipe Directions
Grill chicken breasts with a light coating of salt and pepper. Prepare your favorite black beans and rice mix as directed. When chicken breasts are finished, slice them horizontally across the breast into thin strips *(think deli slices)*. In a bowl or on a plate, portion out desired amount of black beans and rice. Lay chicken breast slices on top of rice. Squeeze fresh lime on top of chicken and rice and serve.

Chef Tips
Add hot sauce to complete the flavor of the dish, if hot sauce is desired and mouth sores are currently not present. Look for salt content on the bag of rice you purchase, especially if you are being sodium conscious as pre-seasoned mixes can have a very high sodium content. The lime must be added last to the dish as the citrus juice will break down in the dish if it is added too early. The purpose of it in this dish is to cut through the weight of the dish, giving it a clean, fresh, tropical taste. You may also serve with cilantro leaves or fresh chopped onions if so desired. The lime in this dish does a fantastic job of cutting through metallic tastes in the mouth.

CHICKEN CACCIATORE

Recipe Description
A classic Italian dish. Fairly popular in Italian restaurants until recently when it was disregarded and categorized as old fashioned. It is characterized by chicken breasts covered in tomatoes and veggies then baked in the oven until it is fork tender.

Tasting Guidelines
Taste is savory, sweet, and a touch of spicy.
Weight is light, but can be balanced with savory and sugar.
Texture is soft.
Good for people with low to moderate treatment side effects.
Emotional response of home cooked Italian goodness.
Best categorized as family style Italian fare.

Ingredients
3 lbs. chicken breast, uncooked and
cut into bite-sized pieces
1 large can tomatoes, diced
4 stalks celery, chopped
4 carrots, chopped
1 yellow onion, diced
8 oz. portabella mushrooms, sliced
1 can corn kernels, drained
1 c. frozen peas
1 zucchini, unpeeled and quartered
2 tbsp. olive oil
1 fennel bulb, sliced into medium strips *(optional)*

Flavor Balancers
½ tbsp. salt
1 c. red wine
½ tbsp. black pepper
3 shakes red pepper flakes
2 tbsp. red wine vinegar
¼ c. sugar

Aromatics
1 bay leaf
1 tbsp. rosemary
1 tbsp. dried oregano
1 tsp. fennel seed

Recipe Directions
Mix all ingredients together in a large mixing bowl. Preheat oven to 375°F. Pour ingredients into large casserole dish. Several dishes may be required. Bake uncovered for about an hour and a half or until sauce naturally thickens. Serve with a side of basmati rice or angel hair pasta tossed in olive oil, pepper, and parmesan.

Chef Tips
The beauty of this dish is that there is no wrong way to make it. The origin of this dish comes from the Italian "Pollo Alla Cacciatore," which means chicken prepared in the style of a hunter. Simplified, we call this hunters-style chicken. The intended expression of this dish is that you would throw whatever you had available, be it wild mushrooms, celery, carrots, or whatever else you could find in nature and cook it all together. Originally this would have been prepared with a whole chicken roasted over an open fire perhaps using a Dutch oven or using some other similar camping style cookware. So when you prepare this dish, feel free to use whatever veggies you have available on hand, and don't beat yourself up about using the exact ingredients for accuracy.

CHICKEN TETRAZZINI

Recipe Description
A delicious, if unauthentic, American-Italian dish. The highlight of this dish is the excessive use of parmesan and the unashamed use of a generous cream sauce. This dish is another one of my family's favorite recipes. It was first brought into our family by my grandparent's neighborhood gourmet club.

Tasting Guidelines
Taste is cheesy, creamy, and savory.
Weight is heavy, but can be balanced with lemon juice or vinegar.
Texture is soft.
Good for people with low treatment side effects.
Emotional response of being warm and loved.
Best categorized as American-Italian.

Ingredients
4 chicken breast, salt & peppered, grilled, and cubed
2 c. parmesan cheese, grated
1 lb. linguine noodles
1 medium yellow onion, diced
8 oz. portabella mushrooms, sliced
1 small jar pimentos
1 c. heavy whipping cream
½ stick butter
4 tbsp. flour

Flavor Balancers
1 tbsp. soy sauce
1 tbsp. black pepper
1 tbsp. red wine vinegar
2 tbsp. sugar

Aromatics
2 tbsp. garlic, minced
1 tbsp. dried oregano

Recipe Directions
Prepare sauce. Melt butter over medium heat in large sauté pan. Add mushrooms, onions, and garlic. Sauté until onions and mushrooms sweat and onions are translucent. Add soy sauce, pepper, red wine vinegar, and sugar. Stir in flour to soak up the excess butter. Whisk in cream. Allow to thicken. Remove from heat. Stir in pimentos and half of the parmesan. In a large mixing bowl, combine cooked noodles, sauce, and chicken, stirring thoroughly. Transfer to a large casserole dish. Cover top with parmesan. Bake together in a 350°F oven until parmesan is golden brown across the top.

Chef Tips
If it doesn't look like there is going to be enough sauce, add milk to stretch sauce out. This is a family recipe so my mom was extremely partial to this recipe. Notice the lack of salt? That's because the parmesan and soy sauce do a great job introducing saltiness to this dish.

CHICKEN TIKKA MASALA

Recipe Description

A classic Americanized Indian dish. It is famous for its use of curry, yogurt as a sauce, and delicious vegetables. This version is not very authentic, but is made so that the average home cook can get a grasp on the flavors and have a new experience.

Tasting Guidelines

Taste is spicy, savory, sweet, and tart with aromatic notes.

Weight is medium, but can be balanced with vinegar, lemon juice, and sugar.

Texture is crunchy chicken and veggies in a medium consistency sauce.

Good for people with low to moderate treatment side effects.

Emotional response of exciting, new flavors.

Best categorized as home cooked Indian goodness.

Ingredients

2 lbs. chicken breast, thinly sliced uncooked

1 large can diced tomatoes

½ red onion, chopped

1 yellow pepper, chopped

1 green pepper, chopped

2 c. Greek yogurt

1 c. heavy cream

cooking oil

Flavor Balancers

kosher salt to taste

1 tbsp. black pepper

½ tsp. cayenne pepper

1 tbsp. red curry powder

1 tbsp. lemon juice

Aromatics

2 tbsp. garlic, minced

Recipe Directions

Heat a large sauté pan to a medium heat. Add 1 tbsp. cooking oil or just enough to lightly grease the bottom of the pan. Add garlic, peppers, onion, and chicken into pan and lightly sauté, stirring frequently to avoid sticking and burning. When chicken is about halfway cooked, add seasonings and half cup of water. Stir vigorously to make sauce. Allow water to reduce and chicken to develop a nice sautéed texture.

When everything in the pan is cooked thoroughly, stir in tomatoes and cover, leaving at medium-heat to simmer for 15 minutes. After tomatoes have lost their bright red color, stir in cream, yogurt, and lemon juice mixing thoroughly. Allow to simmer at least 15 minutes to allow all flavors to meld together. Taste for flavor, adjusting seasonings as necessary. Should be sweet, spicy, savory, and have a nice, mellow curry flavor. Serve with basmati rice and pitas or naan bread.

Chef Tips

Use Greek yogurt for a more authentic flavor, but be prepared to add honey or sugar as Greek yogurt tends to be very tart. Lemon juice lightens the dish and bonds all the flavors together. This dish is very flavorful and has a nice heat and warmth, but the yogurt and cream really tone down the spiciness of the dish. It is sure to be an instant classic.

CHICKEN POT PIE CASSEROLE

Recipe Description
This recipe is for what I consider to be the easiest way to make a chicken pot pie. The biscuit dough on top adds a nice deviation from the standard flavorless pie crust and makes it fun to eat. The best thing about this dish is it tastes even better as leftovers.

Tasting Guidelines
Taste is savory and hearty.
Weight is medium-heavy, but can be balanced with savory, vinegar, and sugar.
Texture is soft.
Good for people with low to moderate treatment side effects.
Emotional response of a dinner your mom would have made.
Best categorized as classic American.

Ingredients
3 chicken breasts, cooked and chopped
½ c. cheddar cheese
6 oz. red potatoes, medium diced
6 oz. carrots, medium diced
1 yellow onion, medium diced
6 oz. peas
6 oz. corn kernels
1 can cream of chicken
1 can cream of mushroom
1-2 c. water
Your favorite baking quick mix prepared for biscuits, but adding 1 tsp. baking soda.

Flavor Balancers
kosher salt to taste
2 tbsp. soy sauce
black pepper to taste
1 tsp. cayenne or red pepper
2 tbsp. apple cider vinegar or red wine vinegar
1 tbsp. sugar, if using red wine vinegar

Aromatics
2 tsp. red curry powder
1 tbsp. ground sage

Recipe Directions
Bake or sauté your chicken breast. While this is going, sauté your veggies together, being careful not to burn them. Add chopped chicken, and sauté until chicken gets a light brown color. Prepare your biscuit dough as directed, making certain to add the baking soda. Once chicken has gotten a little golden brown on it. Add your spices and seasonings except for soy sauce, vinegar, and sugar. After mixing seasonings thoroughly, add the soy sauce and coat all food thoroughly. Allow soy sauce to reduce. Add vinegar allow to reduce. Add sugar and canned soups. Mix well. If needed, add water to adjust thickness. Add cheddar cheese mixing thoroughly. Pour filling mixture into a large casserole dish, preferably glass or ceramic dish. At this point, it is all personal preference.

Method 1
Roll out biscuit dough into a long sheet of dough. Place sheet of dough over filling, making certain that the dough is larger than the casserole dish. Cut off excess trimmings. Cut small cuts in dough to allow pot pie to vent while cooking.

Method 2

The "drop biscuit" method. This is my preferred method because I feel that it adds a certain southern charm to it. You take the biscuit dough and either roll out the dough onto a sheet and cut biscuits, laying the biscuits on top of the filling -or- free form balls of dough with your hands, about the size of a golf ball, and dot the top of the pot pie filling with freshly made drop biscuit dough. Bake in preheated oven at 375°F until biscuits/pie covering are thoroughly cooked, about 15 minutes.

Chef Tips

If you are in a hurry, and time is of the essence, feel free to save some time and pick up pre-made biscuit dough from your grocery store.

LASAGNA (BAKED)

Recipe Description
A classic Italian dish famous the world over for its layered pasta with delicious filling.

Tasting Guidelines
Taste is savory, cheesy, and meaty.
Weight is heavy, but can be balanced with vinegar and sugar.
Texture is soft.
Good for people with low to moderate treatment side effects.
Emotional response of home cooked goodness.
Best categorized as classic Italian.

Ingredients
1 lb. ground Italian sausage, cooked and browned *(like prepared for tacos)*
1 lb. lean ground beef, cooked and browned *(like prepared for tacos)*
16 oz. mozzarella cheese, shredded
16 oz. ricotta cheese
8 oz. feta cheese
2 oz. parmesan cheese, grated
1 box lasagna noodles
marinara, follow recipe in this book **page 302**
1 green bell pepper, chopped
1 red bell pepper, chopped
1 lb. fresh spinach
1 c. olive oil

Flavor Balancers
1 tbsp. black pepper
1 tbsp. lemon juice
1 tbsp. sugar

Aromatics
2 tbsp. garlic, minced
1 tbsp. Italian flat leaf parsley, chopped

Recipe Directions
Prepare lasagna noodles as directed in well-salted water. Drain noodles. Spray noodles down with cold water to stop the cooking process. Cover well with olive oil. Transfer to container and set to the side.

Ricotta, Feta, Spinach Filling
In a large sauté pan over medium heat, sauté garlic and the red and green peppers until garlic is light brown. Immediately, add fresh spinach. Use a flipping/folding method, wilt the spinach. As soon as spinach is wilted, remove from heat and pour into a mixing bowl. Add ricotta, feta, black pepper, salt, sugar, vinegar, lemon juice, and parsley into mixing bowl. Using a large spoon, mix and mash all ingredients together until all ingredients are blended together well. Set mixture to side.

Assembly

Grease a large casserole pan with olive oil. Place a thin layer of marinara on the bottom of the pan followed by one layer of lasagna noodles. Spread a thin layer of the ricotta mixture on top of the noodles, taking care not to rip them. Place another layer of lasagna noodles on top. Apply a thin layer of marinara and sprinkle ground beef and sausage. Repeat this layering technique until there are no more noodles left, making certain to use all ingredients and to do each layer fairly evenly. The thickness of your layers is determined by the size of your pan. So adjust as you go, using your best judgment. When you reach your final top layer of noodles, cover with a healthy layer of marinara, making certain to not leave any dry spots what so ever and getting it down into the edges as well. Cover the marinara with a healthy sprinkling of mozzarella and parmesan cheese.

Place assembled lasagna in oven and bake at 325°F. About 2 hours or until center has reach 145°F. If the center of the lasagna reaches 145°F. before the cheese starts to brown, simply turn on the broiler and broil on low to finish, taking care not to burn. When done baking, top with fresh Italian parsley.

LINGUINE WITH PEPERONATA

Recipe Description
A surprisingly light pasta dish. Fabulous for summers on the back porch. This dish is characterized by its peppers and sausage and goes especially well with a glass of Chianti.

Tasting Guidelines
Taste is savory and sweet.
Weight is light, but can be balanced with vinegar and red wine.
Texture is soft.
Good for people with low to moderate treatment side effects.
Emotional response of sitting on the Italian Riviera enjoying a good meal and a glass of wine.
Best categorized as Italian.

Ingredients
1 lb. linguine noodles
1 c. peperonata, follow recipe in this book **page 236**
1 c. marinara, follow recipe in this book **page 302**
¼ lb. Italian sausage
¼ c. red wine, for deglazing pan

Recipe Directions
Prepare peperonata and marinara according to their recipes in this book. In a large pan, brown the sausage on medium-high heat, taking care to drain excess grease. After sausage has been drained, mix in peperonata and bring to temperature. Add red wine to deglaze pan. After red wine begins to reduce, stir in marinara and reduce to a medium-low heat. Allow marinara to come to proper temperature with out burning it. Boil linguine noodles in water that is as salty as the ocean. When done, drain noodles well. Toss in sauce, coating evenly. Serve with crusty bread, parmesan, or ricotta salata.

Chef Tips
Make sure that you drain the sausage grease well. The dish is supposed to be light in weight and flavor. If you do not have previously made peperonata, you can make in the same pan as the sausage, after the sausage has been browned and drained of excess grease.

LONDON BROIL

Recipe Description
A culinary classic. London broil is a specific cut of beef that when done incorrectly is like trying to eat a hockey puck. But when done correctly, it is a tender and flavorful steak and is affordable enough to feed the whole family. The key is to never over cook it and to always cut the steak at a 45-degree angle.

Tasting Guidelines
Taste is savory and meaty.
Weight is medium, but can be balanced with salt and rosemary.
Texture is firm and steak like.
Good for people with low to moderate treatment side effects.
Emotional response of a delicious steak dinner.
Best categorized as classic American. Definitely not British.

Ingredients
1 London broil (usually 2-3 lbs.)
2 tbsp. olive oil

Flavor Balancers
kosher salt
meat tenderizer
black pepper

Additional
broiling pan
1 gallon storage bag

Aromatics
1 tbsp. garlic, minced
2 tbsp. fresh rosemary leaves

Recipe Directions
Lightly tenderize meat on both sides with a tenderizing mallet. Take extra time to make certain that the large, hard, fat vein is worked/tenderized extra well. Loosely cover meat with salt, black pepper, and meat tenderizer. Place meat to the side and allow to rest. Take rosemary leaves and smash them with the flat side of your knife. Take a small bowl and add together smashed rosemary leaves, garlic, and olive oil, mixing together well. Apply mixture to front and back of London broil then place inside of large storage bag. Allow to marinate on the counter for 30-45 minutes.

Now from here there are two ways you can cook the London broil:

Easy Method
Preheat the oven to 275°F. Place on a broiling pan. Put in the oven and allow to cook until internal temperature reaches 125°F, which is medium rare. Pull out immediately. Allow to rest 15 minutes before slicing. Slice along the shortest end of the steak at a 45-degree angle, creating thin long strips. Serve as desired.

Advanced Method
Take a large cast iron skillet. Heat it as hot as you can on the stove. Sear meat for 3 minutes on

each side. Immediately remove from heat using a thermometer to check internal temperature for 125°F. If London broil is not at temperature, return to skillet and sear in 30-60 second increments until desired temperature is reached. Remove from heat and allow to rest at least 15 minutes before cutting. Slice thin slices at a 45-degree angle starting at the thinnest side of the steak.

Chef Tips

Allowing the meat to rest before carving; it makes the meat more juicy. The reason you let the London broil marinate at room temperature on the counter versus at forty degrees in the refrigerator is quite simply that when you expose cold meat to heat, the outside cooks dramatically faster than the inside of the meat. What happens is the outside meat becomes over-cooked, while the inside is still not done. By the time this is finished it will be a tough piece of meat. Raising the internal starting temperature, even 30 degrees to room temperature, allows for the outside of the meat to cook at the same rate. This also allows the internal temperature to raise equally, leading to a more tender piece of meat in the end. On a London broil, which is already tough to start with, we want to do everything we can to reduce toughness. Also, we want to let the London broil rest at room temperature because there are little enzymes in the meat that will break down the tougher parts resulting in a more tender meat. They only work at warmer temperatures under 120°F. This has been proven through food science and the preparation technique known as sous vide. In this recipe, it might be prudent to finish the chemo patient's London Broil in a sauté pan after cooking, allowing it to raise to a well done temperature of 151°F to prevent food borne illness.

MAC N CHEESE (BAKED)

Recipe Description
A classic casserole dish from the 1950's. This dish is characterized by its ease of preparation and savory, cheesy flavor.

Tasting Guidelines
Taste is savory and cheesy with a hint of salty.
Weight is heavy, but can be balanced with vinegar.
Texture is soft.
Good for people with low to moderate treatment side effects.
Emotional response of childhood memories.
Best categorized as comfort food.

Ingredients
4 slices bacon, cooked and chopped
1 lb. elbow macaroni, cooked in salted water
8 oz. sharp cheddar, shredded
8 oz. American cheddar, shredded
½ yellow onion, chopped
1 c. milk
1 tbsp. butter
1 tbsp. flour

Flavor Balancers
1 tsp. kosher salt
½ tbsp. black pepper
1 tsp. red pepper flakes
1 tbsp. red wine vinegar
½ tbsp. sugar

Aromatics
1 tbsp. garlic, minced
1 tbsp. bay seasoning

Recipe Directions
Preheat your oven to 375°F. In a large sauce pan, melt butter over medium heat. Add onion and garlic. Allow onions to caramelize stirring frequently. Stir in flour until butter is absorbed. Add milk. Stir thoroughly, avoiding burning the milk. Add seasonings and cheese. Mix thoroughly, and taste for flavor. Slowly stir in cooked macaroni. If there is not enough sauce, slowly add milk until pasta is thoroughly coated. Adjust seasonings as necessary. Bake in deep casserole dish at least 15 minutes.

Chef Tips
To make this more of a meal, add some cooked, cubed chicken breast. This is a fantastic meal in itself or used as a side.

MOSTACCIOLI (BAKED)

Recipe Description
Baked mostaccioli is a native dish to St. Louis, Missouri. It is our version of Chicago's baked ziti except we use mostaccioli or penne noodles instead, giving the dish a completely different texture. In this dish, pasta is tossed in the sauce, covered with cheese, and baked in the oven until the cheese is perfectly melted. What makes this dish great is that the sauce bakes into the noodles, giving it a completely different flavor.

Tasting Guidelines
Taste is savory, meaty, and cheesy.
Weight is heavy but can be balanced with spicy, vinegar, and sugar.
Texture is soft with occasional crunch.
Good for people with low to moderate side effects.
Emotional response of a good Italian meal.
Best categorized as family style Italian food.

Ingredients
1 lb. ground turkey, 90/10 lean ground beef, or Italian sausage, browned with grease drained
1 c. parmesan cheese, shredded
1 lb. fresh mozzarella, sliced into thin circles
1 box penne or mostaccioli, cooked
1 yellow onion, chopped and sautéed
marinara, follow recipe in this book **page 302**

Flavor Balancers
1 tsp. kosher salt
½ tbsp. black pepper

Aromatics
1 tbsp. garlic, minced
½ tbsp. dried oregano
4 fresh basil leaves, chopped

Recipe Directions
Preheat oven to 375°F. Move fresh mozzarella and fresh basil to the side. Combine all remaining ingredients in a large mixing bowl, making certain to mix all ingredients thoroughly. Pack mixture into suitably sized casserole dish. Cover with fresh mozzarella slices, and bake until mozzarella is thoroughly melted and center of casserole has reached 145°F. Remove from oven, garnish with fresh basil, and serve with parmesan cheese and crusty bread.

Chef Tips
If you live in the Saint Louis area and have the opportunity, substitute the fresh mozzarella for provel. You'll thank me later. You can also use any kind of tasty, melty cheeses like Gruyère, taleggio, or ricotta salata. I highly recommend getting a hold of some high quality pecorino romano and hand grating it in place of the parmesan.

PASTA ALLA MARCO

Recipe Description
Pasta alla Marco is a fun and sassy pasta dish that adds variety to everyday pasta. Its bright color and fun textures make eating pasta fun and delicious.

Tasting Guidelines
Taste is savory, sweet, and a little spicy.
Weight is light to medium, but can be balanced with vinegar and sugar.
Texture is soft and crunchy.
Good for people with low to moderate treatment side effects.
Emotional response of summer time fun.
Best categorized as modern Italian cuisine.

Ingredients
4 oz. spicy salsiccia
1 box bow tie pasta
1 can diced tomatoes
½ red onion, cut into thin strips
1 red pepper. seeded and cored, cut into thin rings, then the rings cut in half
1 tbsp. olive oil
parmesan, optional

Flavor Balancers
1 tsp. kosher salt
1 c. red wine
½ tbsp. black pepper
2 tbsp. red wine vinegar
2 tbsp. sugar

Aromatics
2 tbsp. garlic, minced
1 tsp. dried oregano

Recipe Directions
In a 2 qt. sauce pan, heat oil to a medium heat. Add sausage, garlic, onion, and red peppers. Sauté until onions are translucent. Add red wine and mix thoroughly. Allow red pepper and onions to soak up the wine. Add salt, black pepper, red wine vinegar, sugar, oregano, and tomatoes. Stir well and cover.

Allow to work on stove top for 45 minutes over medium heat, stirring every few minutes to avoid burning the tomatoes. Ten minutes before sauce is finished, prepare noodles in well-salted water. Prepare pasta as directed on box. Do not allow to over cook. Drain pasta and lightly cover with olive oil, mixing to avoid sticking. Return pasta to pot, making sure not to place the pot back on the hot burner. At this point, you want to taste the sauce; add extra sugar if it's too acidic. After sauce is satisfactory, toss pasta with sauce and serve.

Chef Tips
Don't be alarmed if the sauce turns out thin with chunks of tomato. This is what we are looking for. Also, cheap, low-quality pastas will be mushy. Get a good quality pasta for a firm texture.

PORK CHOPS WITH DRIED PLUM SAUCE (GRILLED)

Recipe Description

A classic Spanish dish, mostly unheard of in the United States. This dish truly is something special and is extremely easy to prepare if you are familiar with the ingredients. The dried plums are also great for digestion with an added benefit as chemotherapy can cause problems in this area.

Tasting Guidelines

Taste is savory and sweet.
Weight is medium but can be balanced with savory and sweet.
Texture of this dish is meaty.
Good for people with low to moderate treatment side effects.
Emotional response of eating a good grilled dinner.
Best categorized as classic Spanish.

Ingredients

6 pork loin chops
8 oz. pitted prunes (dried plums)
1 c. water
2 tsp. cornstarch

Aromatics

1 sprig of rosemary
1 tsp. cinnamon

Flavor Balancers

1 tsp. kosher salt
½ c. red wine
2 tsp. ground black pepper
1 tbsp. red wine vinegar
1 tbsp. sugar

Recipe Directions

Salt and pepper the pork chops on front and back. Allow to rest at room temperature for 30 minutes before grilling.

In a medium sauce pan, combine the prunes, cinnamon, salt, black pepper, red wine, rosemary, and water. Bring to a boil until prunes have re-hydrated. Then, using a whisk, mash the prunes until they have become more liquefied and mix well. Add 1 tbsp. of red wine vinegar and sugar. Whisk well and allow to simmer for 5-10 minutes. Taste sauce and adjust seasonings as necessary. Sauce should taste like savory sugared plums with a bit of dryness on the back. Add cornstarch as necessary to thicken. When pork chops are finished grilling, serve with sauce over and under.

Chef Tips

This dish is amazing! Not only are grilled pork chops amazing, but the dried plum sauce adds a whole new level of enjoyment to the pork chops. Prunes are also packed with potassium, B12, B6, fiber, and an enzyme that helps re-hydrate your intestines, making it easier to go to the bathroom. Don't be afraid of this dish because of the prunes. The added sugar and cinnamon really livens it up. And you will be glad you ate this! This recipe is also great for people who are getting backed up and bloated. This dish is a great all natural way to help get things moving along. *Wink*

PORK LOIN WITH ORANGE SAUCE

Recipe Description

A surprisingly wonderful combination. The unique flavor of the pork combined with the natural sweetness of the oranges highlights the naturally sweet and savory character of the pork, creating a surprisingly light and delicious meal.

Tasting Guidelines

Taste is sweet and savory.

Weight is light, but can be balanced with sugar.

Texture is meaty.

Good for people with low to moderate treatment side effects.

Emotional response of a delicious roasted meal.

Best categorized as Mediterranean.

Ingredients

1 pork loin, at least 2 lbs. in weight

2 oranges

Aromatics

1 tsp. ground ginger

Flavor Balancers

kosher salt to taste

2 tbsp. light soy sauce

1 tbsp. dark soy sauce

black pepper to taste

2 tsp. red pepper flakes

1 tbsp. red wine vinegar

1 c. orange juice

1 c. sugar

Recipe Directions

Season pork loin across all surfaces with salt and pepper. Allow to rest on counter for at least 30 minutes at room temperature before baking.

In a medium sauce pan, combine orange juice, red pepper flakes, dark and light soy sauce, red wine vinegar, and ginger. Bring to a medium heat. Allow to simmer 10 minutes. Take one orange and cut in half. Squeeze fresh juice from both halves into sauce, taking care to strain the seeds. Place orange rind into sauce. Allow to simmer 10 additional minutes.

Remove rind. Slowly whisk in sugar. Taste for sweetness. When sauce is sweet, pour over pork roast and bake in oven at 375°F. until internal temperature reaches 145°F. Slice and serve with fresh orange slices as garnish.

POT ROAST

Recipe Description
Pot roast is an American classic found everywhere from restaurants to the frozen food isle. It is comprised of a slow cooked chunk of meat, suspended in liquid, and surrounded by vegetables and potatoes.

Tasting Guidelines
Taste is warm, savory, hearty, and filling.
Weight is heavy, but can be balanced with vinegar.
Texture is soft.
Good for people with low to moderate chemotherapy side effects.
Emotional response of home-cooked love.
Best categorized as a comfort food.

Ingredients
2 lbs. chuck roast
(use round roast if less-fatty meat is desire)
3 carrots, chopped
1 yellow onion, quartered into wedges
(think like Chinese food)
6 small red potatoes, quartered
3 celery stalks, chopped
1 c. water
2 small cans beef consume
1 tbsp. cornstarch

Flavor Balancers
kosher salt to taste
black pepper to taste
2 tbsp. red wine vinegar
2 tbsp. sugar

Aromatics
2 tbsp. garlic, minced
2 bay leaves
1 sprig fresh rosemary

Recipe Directions
Start with the rosemary. Using a large chef's knife on a cutting board of suitable size, utilize the flat part of the blade to crush and drag the rosemary needles. Doing this will release more of its fantastic oil, creating an extremely aromatic dish.

Next, cover all surfaces of the roast with salt and pepper. Bring a large skillet to high heat. Take roast and brown all sides of roast. Allow it to cook until each side gets a nice char on it. When all sides are sufficiently brown, transfer into a large slow cooker. Add remaining ingredients. Cook on high about four hours or for a slower cook method, cook on low 8-10 hours until meat is tender and falls apart. After roast is tender, slice for serving when appropriate.

Chef Tips
Use beef round instead of chuck, if it is difficult for heavier foods to be kept down. A chuck roast is fattier and therefore will yield a more tender finished product. This is why it is usually recommended.

My favorite part about this recipe is that it is actually two dishes in one. Whatever you have that is leftover can be left in the pot and additional veggies can be added. Just add more soup base or water and cook over night on low to have a wonderful beef stew in the morning!

If pot roast is too heavy, add red wine vinegar. Don't be afraid to add a healthy dose of sugar to make the pot roast more appealing to your loved one.

A couple of dashes of red pepper flakes really fill out this recipe, hitting all of those flavor senses.

RATATOUILLE

Recipe Description
A classic southern French dish often categorized as a peasant food because of its low cost and lack of meat in the dish. Made famous by the movie of the same name, this dish is indeed fantastic.

Tasting Guidelines
Taste is savory.
Weight is light, but can be balanced with savory.
Texture of this dish is soft.
Good for people with low to moderate treatment side effects.
Emotional response of home cooked love.
Best categorized as classic French.

Ingredients
1 medium eggplant
1 lb. zucchini, quartered
2 green bell peppers, cut into strips
1 red bell pepper, cut into strips
1 large can tomatoes, diced
2 large red onions, sliced
½ c. olive oil

Flavor Balancers
kosher salt *(lots of it)*
2 tbsp. dark soy sauce
black pepper to taste
2 tbsp. red wine vinegar
2 tbsp. sugar

Aromatics
2 tbsp. garlic, minced
1 whole bay leaf
1 tbsp. dried oregano
2 tbsp. Italian flat leaf parsley, chopped
1 tbsp. fresh basil leaves, chopped

Recipe Directions
The very first step in this recipe is to do what I call "defunking" the eggplant. Eggplant is a naturally bitter food. So to avoid this, we have to do a small amount of additional prep to remove the funkiness and end up with a delicious savory product.

Slice the eggplant into quarter inch thick circles. Then take a colander and line it with paper towels. Sprinkle a little bit of salt on the paper. Now pick up our first slice of eggplant and sprinkle salt on both sides. Lay it down in colander. Pick up your second slice of eggplant and repeat salting method and lay on top of previous placed eggplant slice. Repeat this method, making layers of eggplant and salting in between each layer as you stack. Allow colander to sit in a sanitized sink for at least 30 minutes while eggplant is defunking.

While eggplant is defunking, preheat oven to 375°F. After 30 minutes, rinse your eggplant thoroughly, and cut the rounds into quarters. Now mix all ingredients into large mixing bowl. Transfer to casserole dish. You may need several. Bake at 375°F until juices from vegetables have baked off and ratatouille has a thick consistency, about 1 hour and 30 minutes. Serve with crusty bread and cheese.

Chef Tips
If you do this in a slow cooker, do not use canned diced tomatoes as there is too much liquid. Use about 6 Roma tomatoes cut into ⅛ wedges. The red and green pepper is non-traditional, but I really enjoy them!

RATATOUILLE (GREEK VERSION)

Recipe Description

Very similar in construction to the French version, but with a Greek twist. It features the addition of bell peppers, Feta cheese, potatoes, and, if you are feeling up to it, chicken. This makes it a much heartier meal.

Tasting Guidelines

Taste is savory and hearty.
Weight is light, but can be balanced with savory.
Texture is soft.
Good for people with low to moderate treatment side effects.
Emotional response of home cooked goodness.
Best categorized as classic home style Greek.

Ingredients

8 oz. feta cheese, crumbled
1 medium oval eggplant
1 lb. zucchini, cut into quarters
1 lb. red potatoes, cubed
1 green bell pepper, sliced into this strips
1 red bell pepper, sliced into thin strips
1 large can tomatoes, diced
8 oz. portabella mushrooms, sliced
2 large red onion, sliced
½ c. olive oil

Optional

2 chicken breast, raw and cubed

Aromatics

2 tbsp. garlic, minced
1 tbsp. dried oregano
2 tbsp. Italian flat leaf parsley, chopped

Flavor Balancers

kosher salt *(lots of it)*
2 tbsp. soy sauce
½ tbsp. freshly ground black pepper
8 shakes red pepper flakes
2 tbsp. red wine vinegar
2 tbsp. sugar

Garnish

bread to serve

Recipe Directions

The very first step in this recipe is to do what I call "defunking" the eggplant. Eggplant is a naturally bitter food. So to avoid this, we have to do a small amount of additional prep to remove the funkiness and end up with a delicious savory product.

Slice the eggplant into quarter inch thick circles. Then take a colander and line it with paper towels. Sprinkle a little bit of salt on the paper. Now pick up our first slice of eggplant and sprinkle salt on both sides. Lay it down in colander. Pick up your second slice of eggplant and repeat salting method and lay on top of previous placed eggplant slice. Repeat this method, making layers of eggplant and salting in between each layer as you stack. Allow colander to sit in a sanitized sink for at least 30 minutes while eggplant is defunking.

While eggplant is defunking, preheat oven to 375°F. After 30 minutes, rinse your eggplant thoroughly, and cut the rounds into quarters. Now mix all ingredients into large mixing bowl. Transfer to casserole dish. You may need several. Bake at 375°F until juices from vegetables have baked off and ratatouille has a thick consistency, about 1 hour and 30 minutes. Serve with crusty bread and cheese.

Chef Tips

If you do this in a slow cooker, do not use canned diced tomatoes, as there is too much liquid. Use about 6 Roma tomatoes cut into ⅛ wedges.

SCALOPPINE (CHICKEN OR PORK)

Recipe Description

Chicken scaloppine, also known as escalope or fritter, is a classic ingredient in many Italian dishes like chicken parmesan, chicken marsala, and chicken saltimbocca. It is characterized by a thin piece of chicken breast that has been butterflied, beat with a mallet, breaded, and deep or pan fried. This should always be served with a tasty and flavorful sauce.

Tasting Guidelines

Taste is savory like fried chicken.
Weight is heavy, but can be balanced with a sauce.
Texture is crunchy.
Good for people with low to moderate treatment side effects.
Emotional response of fried chicken on a Sunday.
Best categorized as classic Italian fare.

Ingredients

5 lbs. chicken breasts
4 eggs
1 c. water
oil for frying
1 c. Italian bread crumbs
1 c. cornstarch
1 c. wheat flour

Flavor Balancers

1 tbsp. black pepper

Aromatics

2 tbsp. Italian seasoning

Recipe Directions

Butterfly chicken breasts by cutting in half horizontally. After butterflying all chicken breasts, take a meat mallet and lightly pound chicken breasts, working from the center out, until they form thin patties. In a mixing bowl, combine all dry ingredients, including seasonings, to make breading. In a large, shallow container, prepare egg wash by whisking eggs with water. Fill a spaghetti pot with 1 qt. frying oil. Bring oil to a medium heat, or bring a sizable deep fryer to 375°F.

Hand bread each chicken breast in this method: 1: cover chicken with breading; 2: dip in egg wash, covering thoroughly; 3: return to breading and thoroughly cover; 4: grab the farthest tip of the chicken breast; 5: lift from breading and slowly place into hot oil; 6: only let go of meat when oil is about ½" from your fingers; 7: allow chicken breasts to cook, flipping them after about 4 minutes.

Do not drop breasts into hot oil! This will cause a splashing, which will burn you! You are far less likely to burn yourself when you slowly introduce the meat into the hot oil by hand, only letting go of the meat after it is almost all in the oil!

You will know when they are cooked as the juices coming from the scaloppine will be clear. Remove from oil and allow to dry in a pan lined with paper towels or newspaper to absorb the extra oil. Keep stored in a warm oven until ready to serve. Try not to stack finished scaloppine on top of each other as they will loose their crispness and become soggy.

Chef Tips

Scaloppine can be used for a variety of things. Chicken Parmesan: cover with marinara and parmesan and bake in the oven. Chicken Marsala: toss in Marsala wine sauce. Or, they can be served with country gravy to make Chicken Fried Steaks. If you intend to prepare them for later use, only half-cook them. You can then freeze them and finish them by spraying with cooking spray and baking in the oven at 450°F until crispy.

Great news! This recipe is also perfect for Pork Scaloppine! Substitute chicken breasts for 5 lbs. thinly sliced pork loin. Pork scaloppine can be used for a variety of things. Pork Parmesan: cover with marinara and parmesan and bake in the oven. Pork Marsala: toss in Marsala wine sauce. Or, they can be served with country gravy to make Chicken Fried Pork Steaks.

SHEPHERD'S PIE (BEEF)

Recipe Description
Beef shepherd's pie is a classic dish from the British Isles. It is typically made with lamb. However, in this recipe, we have substituted with lean ground beef for ease of preparation, weight, and flavor palate. Lamb is fatty and heavy, making it a poor choice during cancer treatments. This dish is a layered casserole with a beef, vegetable, and gravy mixture comprising the filling and mashed potatoes layered on top.

Tasting Guidelines
Taste is savory and hearty.
Weight is heavy, but can be balanced with vinegar.
Texture is soft.
Good for people with low to moderate side effects.
Emotional response of warm lovey goodness.
Best categorized as a comfort food.

Ingredients
1 lb. lean ground beef
1 lb. frozen veggie mix
(or your choice of chopped fresh veggies)
2 packs brown gravy mix
(prepared according to directions)
1 tbsp. cooking oil
mashed potatoes,
follow recipe in this book **page 219**

Flavor Balancers
½ tbsp. black pepper
1 tbsp. red wine vinegar
1 tbsp. sugar

Aromatics
1 tbsp. garlic, minced

Recipe Directions
Preheat oven to 425°F. In a large but high-sided sauté pan, bring oil to medium heat. Add ground beef and garlic together. Cook ground beef, constantly chopping it to make small pieces. Add black pepper to taste. After beef has been sufficiently browned, add veggies and a ¼ c. of water. Increase heat to medium-high, allowing vegetables to steam lightly while stirring constantly. When veggies are thoroughly cooked, add brown gravy, mixing thoroughly. The key here is to have gravy coating everything, but to not have the food swimming in the gravy.

Chef Tips
Get a large icing bag. If you do not have one, you can make one out of a one-gallon storage bag by cutting a quarter inch off one of the bottom corners. Fill the bag with potatoes that are warm, but not scalding hot. Pipe mashed potatoes like frosting, in a snake-like motion, back and forth, over the entirety of the top of the dish until all corners are covered. Fill bag with potatoes as necessary. Lightly spray potatoes with cooking spray and place in oven until potatoes are thoroughly toasted. You will know at this point whether you mixed the gravy at the proper proportion or not. If gravy rises up

and bubbles though the potatoes to form lakes of gravy, you have put in too much gravy. If lakes of gravy do not form, then you have used the proper amount of gravy.

SHEPHERD'S PIE (CHICKEN)

Recipe Description
Chicken shepherd's pie is my personal take on the classic dish. It's very similar in construction to the classic shepherd's pie, but it uses chicken in a cream sauce instead of ground beef in a brown gravy. You get the same comforting notes that you get with a regular shepherd's pie but with a twist.

Tasting Guidelines
Taste is savory with aromatic herb notes.
Weight is medium, but can be balanced with spicy and savory.
Texture of this dish is soft.
Good for people with low to moderate treatment side effects.
Emotional response of a good home cooked meal.
Best categorized as a comfort food.

Ingredients
1 lb. chicken breast, cooked and cut into ½" cubes
1 c. sharp cheddar cheese, shredded
1 lb. frozen veggie mix
(like a 4-in-1, small diced veggies)
1 small can cream of mushroom
1 small can cream of chicken
1 tbsp. cooking oil
mashed potatoes,
follow recipe in this book **page 219**

Flavor Balancers
1-2½ tbsp. black pepper
1 tbsp. red wine vinegar
½ tbsp. sugar

Aromatics
1 tbsp. garlic, minced
1 tsp. rosemary
1 tsp. thyme
1 tsp. sage, ground

Recipe Directions
Preheat oven to 425°F. In a large but high-sided sauté pan, bring oil to medium heat. Add cubed chicken breast and garlic together. Cook until chicken develops a little browning on all sides. Add black pepper to taste. After chicken has been sufficiently browned, add veggies and a quarter cup of water increase heat to medium-high, allowing vegetables to steam lightly while stirring constantly. When veggies are thoroughly warmed, add canned soups, cheese, and remaining seasonings, mixing thoroughly. The key here is to have gravy coating everything, but to not have the food swimming in the gravy. Reduce liquid if necessary.

Pick a suitable casserole dish made out of either glass or ceramic. You can choose the depth of the dish. So for example if you prefer an equal mixture of potatoes and filling, use a larger, shallower dish. If you prefer more filling to potato, use a smaller, deeper dish.

Get a large icing bag. If you do not have one, you can make one out of a one-gallon storage bag by cutting a quarter inch off one of the bottom corners. Fill the bag with potatoes that are warm but not scalding hot. And pipe like frosting, in a snake-like motion, back and forth, over the entirety of dish until all corners are covered. Fill bag with potatoes as necessary. Lightly spray potatoes with cooking spray and place in oven until potatoes are thoroughly toasted. About 30 minutes. You will know at this point whether you mixed the gravy at the proper proportion or not. If gravy bubbles though the potatoes, you have put in too much gravy. If lakes of gravy do not form, then you have used the proper amount of gravy.

SPAGHETTI ALA BOLOGNESE

Recipe Description
Very simply translated: spaghetti in the style of the Bolognese. The Bolognese are famous for their meat sauce. And it is fabulous over spaghetti.

Tasting Guidelines
Taste is savory and sweet.
Weight is medium, but can be balanced with vinegar or lemon juice.
Texture of this dish is soft and noodley.
Good for people with low to moderate treatment side effects.
Emotional response of a hearty Italian meal.
Best categorized as classic Italian.

Ingredients
2 lbs. thick spaghetti noodles
marinara, follow recipe in this book **page 302**
1 lb. Italian sausage, ground

Flavor Balancers
kosher salt

Recipe Directions
Brown the sausage in a pan. Drain the grease. Stir sausage into the marinara sauce. Allow to simmer for 30 minutes on a low heat. Allow all flavors to work together.

Boil noodles in water that tastes as salty as the ocean. Toss noodles in sauce, mixing well. Serve with parmesan and crusty bread. Enjoy.

SPAGHETTI ALLA CARBONARA

Recipe Description
A classic Italian Favorite. This dish has been Americanized by utilizing bacon *(smoked cured pork belly)* instead of pancetta *(unsmoked pork belly)* or guanciale *(pork jowl)*, as would be used traditionally in Italy. This dish is a favorite in both America and Italy. And like all true Italian dishes, its brilliance is only matched by its simplicity. The single most difficult part of this dish is ensuring that the heat from the noodles cooks the egg sauce, not the heat from the pan. If done correctly, the egg sauce will bake into the noodles, trapping the pepper and the cheese against the noodle and leaving a dry, baked-on sauce.

Tasting Guidelines
Taste is peppery, cheesy, and savory.
Weight is heavy, but can be balanced with Italian flat leaf parsley.
Texture is dry and noodley.
Good for people with low treatment side effects.
Emotional response of a good Italian meal at a fancy Italian restaurant.
Best categorized as authentic Italian.

Ingredients
8 oz. bacon, chopped into ¼" strips
4 eggs
8 oz. parmesan cheese, grated
1 lb. spaghetti, thick or linguine noodle

Flavor Balancers
2 tbsp. black pepper

Garnish
Italian flat leaf parsley

Recipe Directions
Bring a large spaghetti pot with well-salted water to a boil. In a large sauté pan, begin to cook bacon over medium heat. When water reaches a boil, add pasta and cook. In a bowl on the side, whisk together parmesan, black pepper, and eggs. When pasta finishes cooking, strain and leave in colander.

Bring bacon pan heat to high; make certain bacon is extra crispy. Toss pasta into bacon pan taking care not to burn the pasta, but to toss the bacon grease and bacon thoroughly through the pasta until even. Once pasta is evenly coated, vigorously whisk egg mixture. Turn off heat from pan. Pour egg mixture on top of pasta and stir vigorously.

The key is to not allow the eggs to cook from the heat of the pan, but from the heat of the pasta itself. If your pan is too hot and your pasta is too cold, you will end up with parmesan scrambled eggs and pasta. If you do it correctly, you will end up with pasta that is perfectly coated with parmesan and black pepper as if it was baked into the pasta from the beginning. When finished, top with Italian flat leaf parsley to help with the weight of the dish.

Chef Tips
This pasta dish can be a little heavy so serve in small portions. Feeling adventurous or on a budget? Substitute bacon ends for traditional bacon for a more substantial and rustic feel.

SPAGHETTI AND MEATBALLS

Recipe Description

What would a cookbook be without a decent recipe for spaghetti and meatballs? My father-in-law, Tony's favorite recipe. When he first had this dish, he was immediately transported back to his childhood. Growing up in an Italian family, he immediately declared that Me-Maw would be very proud! This is also one of my mom's favorite dishes and something she asked for weekly when she was going through chemo treatments. Jarred Sauce? FUHGEDDABOUDIT! *(Throw up hands in the air!)* Don't be chintzy! Make my marinara recipe in this book! Take the time and do it right!

Tasting Guidelines

Taste is savory and sweet.
Weight is medium, but can be balanced with lemon juice.
Texture is meaty and noodley.
Good for people with low to moderate treatment side effects.
Emotional response of a good family meal.
Best categorized as Italian.

Ingredients

2 lbs. thin spaghetti noodles, medium bodied
marinara, follow recipe in this book **page 302**
cooking spray
olive oil
kosher salt *(for the boiling water)*

Flavor Balancers

½ tbsp. kosher salt
½ tbsp. black pepper
2-4 shakes crushed red pepper
2 tbsp. lemon juice
2 tbsp. red wine vinaigrette dressing

Meatball Ingredients

1 lb. pork, ground or 1 lb. spicy salsiccia
1 lb. 90/10 lean ground beef
1 c. grated parmesan cheese
2 eggs
bread crumbs as needed

Aromatics

2 tbsp. garlic, minced
1 tbsp. dried oregano
½ tbsp. fennel seed *(optional)*

Recipe Directions

Mix all of the above meatball ingredients, flavor balancers, and aromatics, in a large bowl. Mix with your hands, thoroughly distributing all ingredients. Mix in bread crumbs as necessary to absorb extra moisture. Cover and allow to rest in refrigerator for at least 2 hours.

Preheat oven to 425°F. After meatball mixture is done marinating, roll by hand into your desired size. I prefer to make mine about the size of a golf ball. Now place into a 9x13 baking dish. Make sure that your dish is well coated with cooking spray. After filling dish with meatballs, spray the top of the meatballs with nice even coat of the same cooking spray. Bake until juices run clear and a little bit of the cheese starts melting out. This will vary based on the size of your meatballs. If they are the golf ball size, about 30-45 minutes. If your meatballs are larger, they will take longer.

During last 15 minutes, cook off your spaghetti. Making sure that the water you use is salted enough to taste like the ocean. Don't over cook your pasta. Strain well and lightly coat with olive oil to avoid sticking.

Chef Tips
Some people cook their meatballs in their sauce. I don't do this as you cannot get a good browning on the meatballs, which reduces the savory flavor of the dish. Another reason to bake the meatballs off in the oven, besides the additional savory characteristics, is you can cook off much of the grease. This contributes to a lighter weight meatball. Remember that lighter dishes are easier for chemo patients to eat. One last reminder, make sure your meatballs are all the same size so that they bake evenly.

Recipe Name	Date and Time Eaten	Rating

Recipe Source	Est. Calories

Ingredients and Seasonings

Describe the Taste?

What did you Like?

What did you NOT Like?

What can you add or subtract?

Describe the Texture	Describe the Smell
Any Complications?	How did this recipe make you feel?

Additional Tasting Notes

Recipe Name	Date and Time Eaten	Rating

Recipe Source	Est. Calories

Ingredients and Seasonings

_____
_____
_____
_____

Describe the Taste?

_____
_____
_____
_____

What did you Like?

_____
_____
_____
_____

What did you NOT Like?

_____
_____
_____
_____

What can you add or subtract?

_____
_____
_____
_____

Describe the Texture	Describe the Smell

Any Complications?	How did this recipe make you feel?

Additional Tasting Notes

_____
_____
_____
_____
_____
_____

Recipe Name	Date and Time Eaten	Rating

Recipe Source	Est. Calories

Ingredients and Seasonings

Describe the Taste?

What did you Like?

What did you NOT Like?

What can you add or subtract?

Describe the Texture	Describe the Smell
Any Complications?	How did this recipe make you feel?

Additional Tasting Notes

Recipe Name	Date and Time Eaten	Rating
Recipe Source		Est. Calories

Ingredients and Seasonings

Describe the Taste?

What did you Like?

What did you NOT Like?

What can you add or subtract?

Describe the Texture	Describe the Smell
Any Complications?	How did this recipe make you feel?

Additional Tasting Notes

Recipe Name	Date and Time Eaten	Rating

Recipe Source	Est. Calories

Ingredients and Seasonings

Describe the Taste?

What did you Like?

What did you NOT Like?

What can you add or subtract?

Describe the Texture	Describe the Smell
Any Complications?	How did this recipe make you feel?

Additional Tasting Notes

Recipe Name	Date and Time Eaten	Rating

Recipe Source	Est. Calories

Ingredients and Seasonings

Describe the Taste?

What did you Like?

What did you NOT Like?

What can you add or subtract?

Describe the Texture	Describe the Smell
Any Complications?	How did this recipe make you feel?

Additional Tasting Notes

Recipe Name	Date and Time Eaten	Rating

Recipe Source	Est. Calories

Ingredients and Seasonings

Describe the Taste?

What did you Like?

What did you NOT Like?

What can you add or subtract?

Describe the Texture	Describe the Smell

Any Complications?	How did this recipe make you feel?

Additional Tasting Notes

SIDE DISHES

CAULIFLOWER SAUTE

Recipe Description
Tender cauliflower tossed in a sweet and savory sauce. This is a modified Chinese recipe made for use in the average American kitchen.

Tasting Guidelines
Taste is sweet and savory.
Weight is light, but can be balanced with vinegar.
Texture is soft with a little crunch.
Good for people with low to moderate treatment side effects.
Emotional response of a refreshing change of pace.
Best categorized as American.

Ingredients
1 head of cauliflower
1 tbsp. olive oil

Flavor Balancers
1 tbsp. soy sauce
½ tbsp. red wine vinegar
1 tbsp. sugar

Aromatics
½ tbsp. garlic, minced

Recipe Directions
Steam the cauliflower until tender. In large sauce pan, heat oil to a medium heat. Sauté garlic to a light golden brown. Next, add cauliflower. Sauté cauliflower with garlic. Add remainder of ingredients and seasonings. Cook water out of sauce. Toss cauliflower in sauce until the sauce adheres to the cauliflower. Serve and enjoy.

CHEESY POTATOES

Recipe Description
An old family recipe. No meal in my family is complete with out these cheesy potatoes. I'll never forget the year when my uncle declared he did not like the cheesy potatoes and had never liked the cheesy potatoes after 30 years of eating them. We were all in shock. The only thought that came to mind was, "How could you not like these?" So now I leave this up to you to decide. Are you pro or anti-cheesy potatoes?

Tasting Guidelines
Taste is savory and cheesy.
Weight is heavy, but can be balanced with vinegar.
Texture is soft with a little crunch on top.
Good for people with low treatment side effects.
Emotional response of a delicious home cooked meal.
Best categorized as classic southern fare.

Ingredients
8 oz. sharp cheddar cheese, shredded
1 bag frozen potatoes O'Brien
½ yellow onion, diced
8 oz. sour cream
1 can cream of mushroom soup

Flavor Balancers
½ tbsp. salt
1 tbsp. black pepper
5 shakes red pepper flakes
½ tbsp. red wine vinegar
2 tsp. sugar

Aromatics
½ tbsp. garlic, minced

Recipe Directions
Preheat your oven to 425°F. In a large mixing bowl, combine all ingredients and seasonings and stir thoroughly. Place contents into 9x13 baking dish. Bake uncovered until all surfaces and edges are golden brown, about 45 minutes to an hour. Remove from the oven and stir well before serving.

CHINESE STICKY RICE

Recipe Description
A modified version of the classic Chinese favorite. The key to this dish really is the Chinese sausage. With its distinct flavor, it cuts through the rice and sets the dish apart.

Tasting Guidelines
Taste is lightly sweet, savory, and aromatic.
Weight is medium, but can be balanced with vinegar and spicy.
Texture is soft.
Good for people with low to moderate treatment side effects.
Emotional response of a home cooked meal from my Chinese family.
Best categorized as Chinese.

Ingredients
4 oz. sweet Chinese pork sausage, thinly sliced
(Cantonese or Taiwanese style)
1 c. sushi grade rice
6 green onions, thinly sliced
2 tbsp. olive oil

Flavor Balancers
2 tbsp. light soy sauce
½ tbsp. black pepper
1 tsp. cayenne pepper
2 tbsp. rice vinegar
1 tbsp. sugar

Aromatics
½ tbsp. 5 spice powder

Recipe Directions
Prepare sushi grade rice as directed in a rice cooker. When finished, remove and place into large mixing bowl. Stir in oil and rice vinegar, mixing thoroughly to coat all surfaces. Allow rice to cool until it is warm. The rice needs to be warm, not hot. Add remaining ingredients and seasonings into bowl with rice. Mix thoroughly and be careful to allow soy sauce to be applied evenly. The best way to do this is to add it in small increments, stirring thoroughly in between.

After rice is thoroughly coated and mixed, transfer rice into a baking dish of your choosing. Cover well with either a lid or tin foil. Bake in oven at 375°F. at least one hour. The longer you bake this dish, the more well-integrated the flavors become. Be careful not to over-bake, as the rice could begin to dry out.

Chef Tips
Remember, soy sauce is salty! Don't over-salt. Do not add additional salt to this dish. Rice as advertised is very sticky and will scoop out with a similar texture to rice crispy treats before they harden into the "treat" part.

CORN CASSEROLE

Recipe Description
Another classic southern style dish. The brilliance of this dish is its simplicity. It is almost as if somebody looked in the cupboard and asked, "I wonder what would happen if I mixed these ingredients together?" Nonetheless, a delightfully delicious and addictive side dish.

Tasting Guidelines
Taste is sweet and savory.
Weight is heavy.
Texture is soft.
Good for people with low to moderate treatment side effects.
Emotional response of a delicious southern style meal.
Best categorized as southern style.

Ingredients
1 c. cheddar cheese, shredded
1 package corn muffin mix, mixed according to directions
1 can creamed corn
8 oz. sour cream

Flavor Balancers
¼ c. sugar

Recipe Directions
Combine all ingredients together in bread pan and bake at 375°F. until golden brown on top and an inserted tooth pick comes out clean. About 30 minutes.

GRANDMAS CAST IRON SKILLET CORNBREAD

Recipe Description
A country style classic. Cooking cornbread in a skillet takes it to a whole new level. The addition of honey and sugar in the cornbread also helps compensate for the dryness that cornbread is typically plagued by.

Tasting Guidelines
Taste is sweet.
Weight is medium, but can be balanced with sugar and butter.
Texture is soft, but mealy.
Good for people with low to moderate treatment side effects.
Emotional response of eating cornbread at your grandma's house.
Best categorized as southern-style cooking.

Ingredients
2 boxes of corn bread mix *(make per box instructions)*
1 stick butter

Flavor Balancers
½ c. sugar
½ c. honey

Recipe Directions
Preheat your oven to 425°F. Place the skillet into the oven for at least 20 minutes to allow it to completely come to temperature. Prepare cornbread mix as directed on the packaging, adding the additional sugar and honey into the mix. Remove iron skillet from oven and immediately pour batter into the heated skillet. Bake at 425°F until cooked thoroughly. When finished, top with real butter and a light sprinkling of sugar.

Chef Tips
Add 2 tbsp. extra liquid to compensate for the extra sugar and honey.

MASHED POTATOES

Recipe Description
These mashed potatoes are exactly as advertised. They are perfect. Not too heavy. Not too light. Perfectly savory.

Tasting Guidelines
Taste is savory.
Weight is medium, but can be balanced with salt.
Texture is soft.
Good for people with low to severe treatment side effects.
Emotional response of a good home cooked meal.
Best categorized as classic American.

Ingredients
2 ½ lbs. yellow potatoes
½ c. cream
2 tbsp. parmesan cheese
½ stick unsalted butter
½ c. sour cream

Flavor Balancers
kosher salt to taste
black pepper to taste

Recipe Directions
Chunk up potatoes into small pieces, leaving the skin on. Boil on high for 35-45 minutes or until tender. Strain water from potatoes. Place potatoes back in pot. Add remaining ingredients. Mash by hand or by a hand mixer to desired consistency.

Chef Tips
If potatoes are too thin, add cornstarch and heat on medium heat until thickened. If potatoes are too thick, add more cream or milk. Salt and pepper to taste. If you don't like potato skins, peel potatoes before boiling.

ROASTED RED POTATOES WITH CHEESE

Recipe Description
Good old-fashioned roasted potatoes with a twist.

Tasting Guidelines
Taste is savory.
Weight is medium, but can be balanced with salt.
Texture is crunchy.
Good for people low to moderate treatment side effects.
Emotional response of "Mmmmm... This is good."
Best categorized as American.

Ingredients
2½ lbs. red potatoes, medium diced
¼ c. parmesan cheese
¼ c. cheddar cheese
¼ c. feta
2 tbsp. olive oil

Flavor Balancers
kosher salt to taste
black pepper to taste
1 tsp. cayenne pepper

Aromatics
½ tbsp. dried garlic

Recipe Directions
Toss all ingredients, except the cheeses, in a big mixing bowl. Bake in preheated oven at 425°F. for about 45 minutes to an hour on a large baking sheet. During the last 10 minutes of cooking, pull potatoes out of oven and sprinkle with parmesan, cheddar, and feta. Place back in oven to finish. Serve and eat.

SPANISH RICE

Recipe Description
Classic Spanish rice not from a box? Yes. You can definitely make Spanish rice at home all on your own with this super easy recipe.

Tasting Guidelines
Taste is lightly savory and aromatic.
Weight is light, but can be balanced with salt.
Texture is soft.
Good for people with low to moderate treatment side effects.
Emotional response of a night out at a Mexican restaurant.
Best categorized as classic Spanish.

Ingredients
1 c. generic long grain white rice
1 small can tomatoes, diced
1 tbsp. olive oil
1½ c. chicken stock

Flavor Balancers
2 tsp. kosher salt
2 tsp. black pepper
2 tsp. chili powder

Aromatics
½ tbsp. garlic, minced
1 tsp. oregano, dried

Recipe Directions
Combine all ingredients in rice cooker and turn on. Mix well before serving.

Chef Tips
If you don't have a rice cooker, go buy one. Right now.

Recipe Name	Date and Time Eaten	Rating

Recipe Source	Est. Calories

Ingredients and Seasonings

Describe the Taste?

What did you Like?

What did you NOT Like?

What can you add or subtract?

Describe the Texture	Describe the Smell

Any Complications?	How did this recipe make you feel?

Additional Tasting Notes

Recipe Name	Date and Time Eaten	Rating

Recipe Source	Est. Calories

Ingredients and Seasonings

Describe the Taste?

What did you Like?

What did you NOT Like?

What can you add or subtract?

Describe the Texture	Describe the Smell

Any Complications?	How did this recipe make you feel?

Additional Tasting Notes

Recipe Name	Date and Time Eaten	Rating
Recipe Source		Est. Calories

Ingredients and Seasonings

Describe the Taste?

What did you Like?

What did you NOT Like?

What can you add or subtract?

Describe the Texture	Describe the Smell
Any Complications?	How did this recipe make you feel?

Additional Tasting Notes

Recipe Name	Date and Time Eaten	Rating
Recipe Source		Est. Calories

Ingredients and Seasonings

Describe the Taste?

What did you Like?

What did you NOT Like?

What can you add or subtract?

Describe the Texture	Describe the Smell
Any Complications?	How did this recipe make you feel?

Additional Tasting Notes

Recipe Name	Date and Time Eaten	Rating

Recipe Source	Est. Calories

Ingredients and Seasonings

Describe the Taste?

What did you Like?

What did you NOT Like?

What can you add or subtract?

Describe the Texture	Describe the Smell
Any Complications?	How did this recipe make you feel?

Additional Tasting Notes

SNACK RECIPES

BABA GHANOUSH

Recipe Description

A Mediterranean classic. A pureed spread made of eggplant. Done correctly, this dish is light, savory, and little spicy. Done incorrectly, this dish is bitter, heavy, and terrifying. It may take you a few times to get this dish right. But when you do, you will come back to it over and over again. Serve this with pitas and some good olive oil and you can transform this into a meal that is perfect for anytime of the day.

Tasting Guidelines

Taste is savory and spicy.
Weight is light, but can be balanced with lemon juice and olive oil.
Texture is soft and creamy.
Good for people low to severe treatment side effects.
Emotional response of "Oh man! Where was this all my life?"
Best categorized as Mediterranean.

Ingredients
2 medium oval eggplants

Aromatics
2 tbsp. garlic, minced
1 tbsp. cumin (preferably roasted cumin)
½ c. tahini (sesame paste)
Italian flat leaf parsley, chopped

Flavor Balancers
kosher salt to taste
juice of 1 lemon

Garnish
pita bread, cut into wedges, or savory cracker or crusty bread
olive oil

Recipe Directions

Rinse eggplants well. Brush with olive oil or spray cooking spray. Bake on baking rack in the middle of oven at 450°F. or roast over grill, preferably charcoal if you have the time. Similar to roasting peppers, we are roasting these until the skin is blackened and can simply be pulled off. We also want the eggplant to be thoroughly cooked.

While eggplant is hot, peel off skin and remove stems. If done correctly, the inside of the eggplant should just kind of slide out. Immediately, salt the eggplant. This will ensure that no bitter flavors transfer into the baba ghanoush. If feeling old school, mash eggplants into mixing bowl by hand. If not, use your handy-dandy food processor to reduce eggplant into a puree or a mash. I personally like to add the cumin and garlic at this point so it has a chance to cook into the hot eggplant, mellowing the flavor. After thoroughly mashed, mix in lemon juice and tahini. Check for thickness and flavor. Should taste warm and feel medium bodied at this point.

At this point, you have two choices: put the paste on the stove at a low heat, cover, and allow flavors to work together. Afterward, chill and serve with a healthy portion of olive oil floated on top. Or if you are happy with it, proceed to serve as is with a healthy dose of olive oil floated on top. Serve with your favorite crusty bread, freshly made pitas, or crunchy snack.

Chef Tips
If paste is very thin and watery, mix in more lemon juice. The lemon juice acts as a thickener. If paste is very thick, add more olive oil.

BRUSCHETTA WITH RICOTTA AND PEACHES

Recipe Description
One of my personal favorite dishes! One of those dishes where its brilliance is only exceeded by its simplicity. This is a classic Italian snack that is perfect any time.

Tasting Guidelines
Taste is sweet.
Weight is light, but can be balanced with oregano.
Texture is creamy and crunchy.
Good for people with low to severe treatment side effects.
Emotional response of delicious simplicity.
Best categorized as Italian.

Ingredients
ricotta
1 loaf bread, Italian, French, or crusty wheat
peach preserves

Flavor Balancers
black pepper to taste
dried oregano

Recipe Directions
Slice bread into 1" thick slices. Spread a healthy coating of ricotta on slices. Sprinkle black pepper on top of ricotta. Now smother ricotta with peach preserves. Sprinkle oregano on top.

Chef Tips
Do each step on all slices before moving to the next step. Can be frozen, but not refrigerated. Refrigeration dries out bread where freezing it preserves it properly. For ease and convenience, you can always use a good sandwich bread that has been lightly toasted. Do not toast bread if mouth sores are present.

CAPRESE SALAD

Recipe Description
A classic Italian favorite. Loved the world over, Known for its many variations and simplicity. This is a dish that is hard not to love, especially when it is warm out. Great as an appetizer or as a meal. You can change the texture and consistency of the dish simply by changing the cuts to the tomatoes and mozzarella. For a fun finger food appetizer, slice and stack like an open-faced sandwich. For a fun family style appetizer, chop the tomatoes and mozzarella into cubes. Toss in the marinade and serve with crusty bread.

Tasting Guidelines
Taste is savory, sweet, and fresh.
Weight is light, but can be balanced with basil and vinegar.
Texture is soft.
Good for people with low to moderate treatment side effects.
Emotional response of yummy summer time freshness.
Best categorized as Italian.

Ingredients
1 lb. fresh mozzarella, sliced
5 medium-sized Roma tomatoes, sliced

Flavor Balancers
kosher salt to taste
black pepper to taste
red wine vinaigrette
Aromatics
fresh whole basil leaves

Recipe Directions
Since this is a fresh recipe, rinse tomatoes and basil thoroughly. Slice tomatoes into sandwich slices about a ¼ inch thickness. Lightly sprinkle salt over the tomatoes slices on both front and back.

Allow to sit at room temperature for 10 minutes. Then marinate tomatoes in large mixing bowl in a generous coating of red wine vinaigrette for at least 30 minutes. While tomatoes are marinating, slice fresh mozzarella into similarly sized servings. Set aside.

Remove basil leaves from stem. Then on a large serving platter, assemble in this method: Tomatoes down first. Cheese down second. A sprinkle of fresh black pepper over the cheese. Add basil leaf to finish. Serve chilled or at room temperature.

Chef Tips
May be refrigerated for several days for quick easy snacks through out the week. I highly recommend if you are going to do this to put the basil on fresh every time you serve. This recipe is more like a finger food and can be made more like a salad by chopping everything into thumb nail sized chunks.

Alternatively, you can substitute the vinaigrette for balsamic vinegar and extra virgin olive oil.

FALAFEL

Recipe Description

Falafel is the meatball of the Levant. It is mostly used on sandwiches, but can also be featured on dinner platters. Due to its construction, it is an excellent meat substitute with the beans being high in protein and iron. Falafel is a food item that you either love or can't stand. Done correctly, each ball should be dense and heavily spiced leading to a very flavorful treat. Done incorrectly, they are crumbly, grainy, and not very enjoyable.

Tasting Guidelines

Taste is savory and aromatic.
Weight is medium, but can be balanced with lemon juice and garlic.
Texture is dense. Crunchy on the outside and soft on the inside.
Good for people with low to moderate treatment side effects.
Emotional response of an exotic meal.
Best categorized as classic Mediterranean.

Ingredients

- 2 small cans chickpeas, drained
- 1 can lima beans, butter beans, great northern beans, cannellini or fava, drained
- 2 eggs, scrambled, but uncooked
- ⅛ tsp. baking soda
- 2 tbsp. olive oil

Flavor Balancers

- 1½ tsp. kosher salt
- freshly ground black pepper to taste
- ½ tsp. cayenne pepper
- 1 tbsp. lemon juice

Aromatics

- 1 tbsp. garlic, minced
- ½ tbsp. red curry powder
- ½ tbsp. ground cumin
- ⅛ c. Italian flat leaf parsley, finely chopped

Recipe Directions

Preheat oven to 425°F. In a large mixing bowl, combine all beans, taking care to mash by hand thoroughly. Then add remaining ingredients, mixing thoroughly. It should resemble hamburger or meatballs in consistency. If too wet, mix in cornstarch or flour to dry. If too dry, add a little water or an extra egg.

Paste should be able to be formed by the hand or an ice cream scooper into balls resembling a meatball. Use a muffin pan. Spray with pan spray. Fill muffin pan ½ inch with falafel mix. Bake about 45 minutes. Bake time depends on the size of the falafel balls. Falafel should be crispy on the outside, but moist on the inside. Adjust cook time accordingly.

HUMMUS

Recipe Description

Ten years ago, people would have looked at you as if you had five heads when you talked about hummus. Now, it is in every grocery store across America. It is a bean paste made from the chickpea aka the garbanzo bean. Hummus is actually the Egyptian word for chickpea. Due to its high protein content, the chickpea is a main food staple in the Mediterranean and Middle East. This recipe is fairly authentic. It is simple to make, yet difficult to master. You can infuse the hummus with garlic, roasted red peppers, olives, ground pistachios, or whatever you really feel like. It is exceptionally versatile, and its limitations are only our imagination. Hummus can be used as a sandwich spread, eaten alone, and has many other uses.

Tasting Guidelines

Taste is lightly savory and a little spicy.
Weight is light, but can be balanced with lemon juice and olive oil.
Texture is creamy.
Good for people with low to severe treatment side effects.
Emotional response of healthy goodness.
Best categorized as classic Mediterranean.

Ingredients

1 large can chick peas aka garbanzo beans
½ c. tahini *(sesame paste)*
olive oil as needed

Garnish

pita bread, cut into wedges, or savory cracker or crusty bread
olive oil

Aromatics

2 tbsp. garlic, minced
1 tbsp. cumin *(preferably roasted cumin)*
fresh Italian flat leaf parsley, chopped

Flavor Balancers

kosher salt to taste
juice of 1 lemon

Recipe Directions

Empty chickpeas into a pot and heat until warm, then drain. If feeling old school, mash chickpeas into mixing bowl by hand. If not, use your handy-dandy food processor to reduce chickpeas into a puree or a mash. I personally like to add the cumin and garlic at this point so it has a chance to cook into the hot chickpeas, mellowing the flavor. After thoroughly mashed, mix in this order: tahini, lemon juice, salt, and olive oil.

What you are doing in this recipe is adding the thickening ingredients first, then adding olive oil to thin hummus to desired consistency. Check for thickness and flavor. Should taste warm and feel medium bodied at this point. If paste is very thin and watery, mix in more lemon juice. The lemon juice acts as a thickener. If paste is very thick, add more olive oil.

At this point, you have two choices: put the paste on the stove at a low heat, cover, and allow flavors to work together. Afterward, chill and serve with a healthy portion of olive oil floated on top. Or if you are happy with it, proceed to serve as is with a healthy dose of olive oil floated on top.

Chef Tips
I highly recommend using canned chickpeas over dried ones as it can make quite a mess. The key here is to balance the lemon and the olive oil as explained in the recipe.

If you are a purest and you have the time, you can use dried chickpeas that you properly prepared, taking care to remove the skins that float off. I personally don't have time so I shortcut as do most people who make hummus at home. Typically, in American grocery stores, garbanzo beans are found in the Mexican or ethnic food aisle of a major chain. This style of bean-based spread, or tapenade, can be made out of any fatty, bean like fava, cannellini, great northern, lima, butter beans, etc. It's fun to experiment and try different ones. Also, hummus can always be made with fun flavors like olives, roasted red peppers, and so on. I personally love to put hummus as a substitute for mayonnaise on turkey and Swiss cheese sandwiches.

MUSHROOMS AND PARSLEY

Recipe Description
This is another one of those dishes where its brilliance is exceeded only by its simplicity. Perfect to eat with some nice, crusty bread. It's light, but savory character will make you wish for lots of sunshine and a cool Mediterranean breeze.

Tasting Guidelines
Taste is light and savory.
Weight is light, but can be balanced with lemon juice and parsley.
Texture is soft.
Good for people low to moderate treatment side effects.
Emotional response of a high-end restaurant appetizer.
Best categorized as Mediterranean.

Ingredients
1 lb. mixed mushrooms, portabella, or white button, pre-sliced
⅓ c. cooking olive oil, not extra virgin or light

Flavor Balancers
kosher salt to taste
freshly ground black pepper to taste
1 tbsp. lemon juice
½ c. white wine *(sweet like Moscato or Riesling)*

Aromatics
1 tbsp. garlic, minced
3 tbsp. Italian flat leaf parsley, finely chopped

Recipe Directions
Wash mushrooms and pat dry with paper towels. Heat oil in large frying pan. Add mushrooms and garlic. Cook over medium heat, stirring often, until lightly browned, about 15 minutes. Do not allow garlic to burn or it will make the recipe very bitter. When mushrooms are done sweating, add white wine to soak up the flavor. Bring mixture to boil and reduce sauce. Add lemon juice, salt, and pepper to taste. Transfer to warmed dish and sprinkle with parsley. Serve hot or at room temperature. Serve with bread.

Chef Tips
While cooking mushrooms, what you are looking for is for them to get quick stewed so they will excrete their flavor. You want to bring out the flavor of mushrooms. So feel free to cook them to death.

PEPERONATA

Recipe Description
A classic Italian dish. It is extremely versatile and can be used in many different ways, such as over pasta, as a condiment on a sandwich, eaten by itself with some crusty bread, served with a grilled salsiccia, and many other pairing options. In this book, I offer a recipe that uses the peperonata over pasta. It is absolutely fantastic!

Tasting Guidelines
Taste is savory and peppery.
Weight is light, but can be balanced with red wine and sugar.
Texture is soft.
Good for people with low to moderate treatment side effects.
Emotional response reminding you of a warm summer day.
Best categorized as Italian.

Ingredients
4 bell peppers red, green, yellow, sliced into thin long strips, think fettuccine noodle
1 large can tomatoes, diced
2 medium red onions, sliced long and thin
2 tbsp. olive oil

Flavor Balancers
kosher salt
1-2 c. red wine *(any kind will do)*
freshly ground black pepper to taste
1-2 tbsp. red wine vinegar
¼ c. sugar

Aromatics
2 tbsp. garlic, minced
1 tbsp. dried oregano

Recipe Directions
In a spaghetti pot, bring oil to medium-low heat. Add garlic, onions, green peppers, and black pepper. You want to sweat them. You want to cook everything until the onions begin to caramelize and the green peppers start breaking down. It is better to go low and slow with cooking temperature for this recipe. Deglaze pan with red wine after onions are caramelized and peppers are broken down. Reduce wine. After wine has been reduced, add tomatoes, dried oregano, and vinegar.

Cook on a medium heat, stirring often to avoid burning, until diced tomatoes break down. You will know when this happens because the tomatoes will look less like tomatoes and more like marinara. I like to use a whisk to mash the tomatoes with while cooking.

After about 45 minutes of cooking the tomatoes, taste the sauce specifically looking for acidity and saltiness. Add ¼ c. of sugar and stir well. Allow to simmer 5 minutes. Taste sauce again. Take note of acidity and saltiness. If sauce is still very acidic, add another ¼ c. of sugar. Repeat this method until sauce is no longer acidic and has a mellow pleasant flavor.

The very last step you do is add salt if required. Only add salt in very small measurements if needed. Do not add salt as you go. Add very small amounts of salt at the very end, using the same simmer, add, taste method.

Chef Tips
Peperonata is great as a snack when served with bread. Peperonata is fantastic over pasta and is good when used as a condiment for meat or sausage sandwiches. At home, I use between 4 and 8 oz. of Italian sausage added to the beginning of this recipe when I use it as a pasta sauce. The only issue with this is, for chemo, sausage can be very heavy. Chemo patients tend to have trouble keeping down heavy foods. One way you can solve this is by buying Italian salsiccia in link form and baking those off separately. Slice them like you would hot dogs for a little kid, and try a little bit at a time. Garnish over the pasta.

PIEROGIES

Recipe Description
One of my mom's favorites and an exceptionally easy snack. The main benefit to this dish is that all you have to do is take them out of the freezer and make them really quick. This dish is easy and quick when you're in a pinch for time.

Tasting Guidelines
Taste is savory.
Weight is medium.
Texture is soft.
Good for people with low to severe treatment side effects.
Emotional response of comfort food.
Best categorized as Polish.

Ingredients
1 package frozen pre-made pierogies
2 tbsp. oil

Recipe Directions
Fill sauté pan halfway with water. Bring to a boil. Then add frozen pierogies. Boil about 6 minutes. Dump water and pierogies into strainer. Bring sauté pan back to high heat. Add 2 tbsp. of oil. When oil is hot, add pierogies and pan fry until browned about 4 minutes.

Chef Tips
Makes a good quick snack. Can be found in Walmart in the frozen food aisle and other major grocery stores. Serve with sour cream or hot sauce. My mom went crazy for these because they were so simple!

PITAS

Recipe Description

Pitas are the simplest form of bread. Pitas are the Eastern Mediterranean equivalent of French bread. They are good with everything. Pitas are good by themselves, served with a spread like hummus or baba ghanoush. With a little extra oil, they are perfect for sandwiches.

Tasting Guidelines

Taste is sweet and savory with yeasty undertones.
Weight is medium.
Texture is soft.
Good for people with low to moderate treatment side effects.
Emotional response of yummy warm bread goodness.
Best categorized as Eastern Mediterranean.

Ingredients

3 c. flour, plus some extra for rolling out
2 tbsp. olive oil or cooking oil is fine
1–2 c. of warm, but not hot water
1 packet yeast
2 tbsp. sugar
1 tsp. kosher salt

Recipe Directions

Activate your yeast as directed on yeast packet. Next, in a large mixing bowl, combine all ingredients except the water. Mix. Add water as necessary until you make a proper bread dough ball. After dough ball is formed, knead about 10 minutes or until bread develops some nice gluten. The dough will start soft, then get firm, then get extremely soft again. At this point, you know that you have kneaded enough. This is when a kitchen mixer is fantastic with a dough hook. Dough should look and feel like bread dough. Not too sticky, not too dry.

If it's too sticky, mix in more flour. If too dry, add more water. Allow to rise in a warm, humid area covered with a moist towel or paper towel to keep it wet or keep it from drying out for at least 3 hours. The longer it rises, the better of a flavor it will develop. Remove dough from bowl. Cut into balls 2-3 inches in diameter. Should make about 8. Allow to rest about an hour.

At this time, take a pizza stone and put it in your oven. Heat as hot as it will go without burning down the house. Heat to at least, 425°F. If you do not have a pizza stone, you should go out and get one. They are about fifteen dollars. You can even order them off the internet. You can also use a baking sheet instead. The idea here is to have a flat, hot surface to shock the dough into cooking.

Roll out one ball of dough. You want it thin, but not paper thin. Paper thin will burn, and if it's too thick it will cook more like a naan bread. The idea here is to get it somewhere between 1-2 millimeters in thickness. If the dough will not stay rolled out in length and begins to contract, roll the dough back into a ball and allow to process longer. Assuming your dough is happy and healthy, what we want to do is throw each pita onto the stone or pan and allow it to cook until it makes a poof, or a pita pocket.

If you did everything correct, this will happen, and you will have a nice light brown pita with a perfect pocket. If you didn't do everything correctly down to the last detail, you will get some nice bubbles throughout the entirety of the dough and a very pliable pita perfect for making sandwiches.

Depending on the temperature of your oven, this process should take about 2-4 minutes. Remember to allow your stone or pan to come back up to temperature in between making pitas. I like to roll them out one by one so I can be certain to hit the correct temperature in between.

Chef Tips
Pitas are very easy to make, but there is a learning curve. Especially when learning when the dough is properly proofed. When pitas are properly proofed, the dough is malleable and easy to work with and will retain the shape you stretch it out to. When improperly proofed, they will be difficult to work with. The other important part of making pitas is to make sure that you knead the dough properly to develop nice long gluten proteins. Otherwise, they will not poof correctly and will be difficult to stretch. Time is the key here. Don't rush the pitas, if they aren't ready just wait and let them work.

With pitas, practice makes perfect. Do not get discouraged if they do not turn out perfectly the first time. This same recipe can be used to make fresh pizza dough! I simply increase the oil from 2 tbsp. to a ½ c. Increasing the oil makes the dough softer and spongier when cooked. It also helps maintain moisture after cooking. This recipe will yield two large pizzas. If you like really crispy pitas or pizza, remove the oil entirely. These pitas are perfect for making sandwiches or serving with dips and tapenades, like hummus or baba ghanoush.

RICOTTA AL FORNO

Recipe Description
This is one of those dishes that you'll be hesitant to try. You will pass it and pass it and pass it. But then one day, you will decide to try it, and your whole world will never be the same. Perfectly creamy, sweet, and savory. This is somewhere between a dessert and an appetizer. After you have this for the first time, you will be kicking yourself that you didn't have it every time.

Tasting Guidelines
Taste is creamy, sweet, and savory.
Weight is medium, but can be balanced with honey and pepper.
Texture is soft.
Good for people with low to moderate treatment side effects.
Emotional response of "Why did I never eat this before?"
Best categorized as classic Italian.

Ingredients
small plastic container of ricotta *(about 8oz)*
1 tbsp. olive oil

Flavor Balancers
black pepper to taste
2 tbsp. honey

Optional
paprika

Recipe Directions
In a mixing bowl, mix all ingredients until consistent. Fill into a pie tin. Bake at 425°F. until cohesive and melty, about 10-15 minutes.

Chef Tips
Tub ricotta is very moist. So if you desire a less moist product and possibly a little bit of toasting, squeeze the extra moisture out of ricotta before preparing. Serve hot or cold. Serve with crusty bread.

SUMMER SALAD

Recipe Description
This salad is absolutely one of my favorites to eat during the summer. The tomatoes and the cucumbers work together to make a dish that is both savory and light. The vinegar in this dish is what really pulls all the flavors together. The longer you let this marinate, the more homogenized the flavors become.

Tasting Guidelines
Taste is savory.
Weight is light, but can be balanced with red wine vinaigrette.
Texture is like a salad.
Good for people with low to moderate treatment side effects.
Emotional response of summer time freshness.
Best categorized as Mediterranean.

Ingredients
8 oz. feta cheese, diced
4 Roma tomatoes
1 large cucumber
2 green bell peppers
1 medium red onion, sliced
Kalamata olives, a generous but reasonable helping

Flavor Balancers
kosher salt to taste
freshly ground black pepper to taste
red wine vinaigrette

Recipe Directions
Rinse all fresh ingredients thoroughly before cutting. Cut all ingredients into 1" chunks. Place prepared ingredients in large serving bowl. Sprinkle with feta cheese and olives. Toss dressing with all ingredients 30 minutes before serving.

TABOULEH

Recipe Description
A classic Mediterranean dish. Traditionally made with cracked burghul wheat. It is a perfectly light side dish. This recipe has been Americanized slightly by substituting couscous for the wheat. But, it still maintains its texture, palate cleansing effects, and pop of freshness. This dish is a perfect palate cleanser. It contains not one, but two types of palate cleansers which are fresh Italian parsley and fresh squeezed lemon.

This recipe is really good for people with a lot of metal taste in their mouth. This is specifically because of the strength and cleansing properties of Italian flat leaf parsley and fresh lemon.

Tasting Guidelines
Taste is fresh and clean.
Weight is super light, but can be balanced with olive oil.
Texture is grainy.
Good for people with low to severe treatment side effects.
Especially good for severe side effects to get rid strong metallic tastes.
Emotional response of a crisp, cool breeze.
Best categorized as Mediterranean.

Ingredients
1 box instant couscous, prepared as directed on box, then chilled
3 green onions
olive oil as needed

Flavor Balancers
1½ tsp. kosher salt
freshly ground black pepper to taste
½ c. fresh lemon juice

Aromatics
3 tbsp. fresh mint, finely chopped
2 c. Italian flat leaf parsley, finely chopped

Recipe Directions
Take cooked and chilled couscous and place in large mixing bowl. Add green onions and parsley. Toss in lemon juice and remaining ingredients. Mix thoroughly until couscous has absorbed all of the lemon juice. Add olive oil 1 tbsp. at a time for a touch of creaminess.

Chef Tips
Best eaten chilled or at room temperature. It is a great snack and goes great with hummus or baba ghanoush on top of pitas or bread. If metal taste is severe in your mouth, increase parsley and lemon juice. Recipe should taste light and refreshing. Traditionally made with cracked burghul wheat, couscous can be used as an acceptable substitute.

½ c. may be too much lemon juice. Taste as you go trying not to completely over power the dish.

Recipe Name	Date and Time Eaten	Rating

Recipe Source	Est. Calories

Ingredients and Seasonings

Describe the Taste?

What did you Like?

What did you NOT Like?

What can you add or subtract?

Describe the Texture	Describe the Smell

Any Complications?	How did this recipe make you feel?

Additional Tasting Notes

Recipe Name	Date and Time Eaten	Rating
Recipe Source		Est. Calories

Ingredients and Seasonings

Describe the Taste?

What did you Like?

What did you NOT Like?

What can you add or subtract?

Describe the Texture	Describe the Smell
Any Complications?	How did this recipe make you feel?

Additional Tasting Notes

Recipe Name	Date and Time Eaten	Rating
Recipe Source		Est. Calories

Ingredients and Seasonings

Describe the Taste?

What did you Like?

What did you NOT Like?

What can you add or subtract?

Describe the Texture	Describe the Smell
Any Complications?	How did this recipe make you feel?

Additional Tasting Notes

Recipe Name	Date and Time Eaten	Rating

Recipe Source	Est. Calories

Ingredients and Seasonings

Describe the Taste?

What did you Like?

What did you NOT Like?

What can you add or subtract?

Describe the Texture	Describe the Smell
Any Complications?	How did this recipe make you feel?

Additional Tasting Notes

Recipe Name	Date and Time Eaten	Rating

Recipe Source	Est. Calories

Ingredients and Seasonings

Describe the Taste?

What did you Like?

What did you NOT Like?

What can you add or subtract?

Describe the Texture	Describe the Smell

Any Complications?	How did this recipe make you feel?

Additional Tasting Notes

Recipe Name	Date and Time Eaten	Rating
Recipe Source		Est. Calories

Ingredients and Seasonings

Describe the Taste?

What did you Like?

What did you NOT Like?

What can you add or subtract?

Describe the Texture	Describe the Smell
Any Complications?	How did this recipe make you feel?

Additional Tasting Notes

Recipe Name	Date and Time Eaten	Rating
Recipe Source		Est. Calories

Ingredients and Seasonings

Describe the Taste?

What did you Like?

What did you NOT Like?

What can you add or subtract?

Describe the Texture	Describe the Smell
Any Complications?	How did this recipe make you feel?

Additional Tasting Notes

Recipe Name	Date and Time Eaten	Rating
Recipe Source		Est. Calories

Ingredients and Seasonings

Describe the Taste?

What did you Like?

What did you NOT Like?

What can you add or subtract?

Describe the Texture	Describe the Smell
Any Complications?	How did this recipe make you feel?

Additional Tasting Notes

Recipe Name	Date and Time Eaten	Rating
Recipe Source		Est. Calories

Ingredients and Seasonings

Describe the Taste?

What did you Like?

What did you NOT Like?

What can you add or subtract?

Describe the Texture	Describe the Smell
Any Complications?	How did this recipe make you feel?

Additional Tasting Notes

SOUP RECIPES

BAKED POTATO SOUP

Recipe Description
Baked potato soup is a lovely dish when you are in the mood for a hearty cup of soup. Very similar in construction to clam chowder. The appeal of baked potato soup is that without the seafood aspect, the dish loses its pungency and becomes more approachable.

Tasting Guidelines
Taste is savory.
Weight is medium, but can be balanced with red wine vinegar.
Texture is soupy.
Good for people with low to moderate treatment side effects.
Emotional response of having a warm full belly.
Best categorized as classic American.

Ingredients
2 c. sharp cheddar cheese, shredded
4 c. potatoes, yellow or red, diced
2 cans whole kernel corn, drained
1 c. carrots, diced
1 c. celery, diced
1 yellow onion, diced
¼ c. green onions, sliced
2 large cans chicken broth
½ c. butter or 2 sticks of butter
4 c. whole milk
½ c. all purpose flour

Flavor Balancers
1 tsp. kosher salt
1 tbsp. black pepper
1 tbsp. red wine vinegar
1 tbsp. sugar

Aromatics
2 tbsp. garlic, minced
2 bay leaves
2 tbsp. bay seasoning

Garnish
crispy bacon & green onions, chopped for garnish
sour cream

Recipe Directions
In a medium sauce pan, melt butter over medium heat. When butter is thoroughly melted, stir in flour until all butter has been absorbed by flour. Stir thoroughly and be careful not to burn. Allow mixture to remain over heat for 30 seconds to cook the flour flavor out. Immediately remove mixture from heat and set to side for later use.

Bring a large stock pot to medium heat and add oil. Then add garlic, celery, onions, and carrots. Cook over medium heat. Allow to cook until onions are translucent. Stir in potatoes, remaining seasonings, and chicken broth. Bring to a boil for 30 minutes or until potatoes become tender. In the microwave, cook the milk until warm, but not boiling. Add to pot after potatoes are tender, making certain to stir in thoroughly. At this point, taste the soup and make any flavor adjustments necessary.

Over medium-high heat, slowly add roux and allow soup to thicken until a desired consistency is reached. This process should happen in 2-3 minute increments.

The method is: Add roux. Stir. Return to simmer while stirring. If after returning to a simmer, the soup has not thickened sufficiently, add roux and repeat process.

After soup is sufficiently thick, turn burner to low heat and slowly stir in cheddar cheese.

Chef Tips

If soup is too heavy, add red wine vinegar. If soup does not feel full in flavor, it's missing sugar. If it doesn't taste savory, add a little MSG. If you are not concerned about color, instead of using MSG, add a little soy sauce instead. Soy sauce will darken the color of the soup.

BEEF STEW (FRENCH)

Recipe Description

What makes French beef stew different from traditional beef stew is the generous use of red wine and the additional sweetness that the dish takes on as a result. Perfect for a cool or cold day or for when you feel like you just need to get a hearty meal into you.

Tasting Guidelines

Taste is savory.

Weight is heavy, but can be balanced with vinegar and sugar.

Texture is soft.

Good for people with low to moderate treatment side effects.

Emotional response of good ole' fashioned comfort food.

Best categorized as classic French.

Ingredients

1 lb. beef round, cut in ½" cubes
4 large carrots, sliced
1 yellow onion, sliced
4 celery stalks, sliced
1 lb. fresh mushrooms
1 lb. small white onions
10 red potatoes, cut into chunks
1 small can diced tomatoes
2 cans beef consommé

Flavor Balancers

kosher salt to taste
2 c. red wine
black pepper to taste

Aromatics

2 tbsp. garlic, minced
1 bay leaf
1 tbsp. rosemary
2 tsp. thyme

Recipe Directions

Combine all ingredients into a large slow cooker and allow to cook on low overnight until the meat falls apart. If liquid is not enough to cover all ingredients, supplement with water to cover all ingredients. After meat begins to fall apart, mix beef thoroughly throughout the dish and serve after proper seasonings have been determined to be satisfactory. Add cornstarch mixture to thicken sauce if required.

CHICKEN AND DUMPLINGS

Recipe Description
Chicken and dumplings is the southern equivalent to chicken noodle soup. When you are sick or you do not feel good, nothing else will do. And nobody will ever make it better than your mom or grandma. But, here is how I made it for my mom when she went through chemotherapy.

Tasting Guidelines
Taste is savory and aromatic.
Weight is medium, but can be balanced with vinegar.
Texture is soft.
Good for people with low to moderate treatment side effects.
Emotional response of a full belly and home cooked love.
Best categorized as southern American.

Ingredients
2 lbs. chicken breast, shredded
1 pack frozen dumplings *(or make from scratch)*
1 bag frozen stew vegetables *(or fresh veggies)*
1 c. cream *(optional)*
2 c. milk
1 large can chicken stock
1 c. water
1 stick butter
½ c. flour

Flavor Balancers
½ tbsp. kosher salt
½ tbsp. black pepper
½ tsp. cayenne pepper
1 tbsp. red wine vinegar
2 tbsp. sugar

Aromatics
2 tsp. rosemary
1 tbsp. bay seasoning
1 tbsp. sage

Recipe Directions
In a large spaghetti pot, melt butter over medium heat. Add stew vegetables and cook until tender. Stir in flour to absorb extra butter. Mix in additional ingredients and seasonings, except dumplings. Allow to simmer 5 minutes to check seasoning levels. When proper seasoning levels have been reached, break and add frozen dumplings, slowly mixing in to avoid sticking. Transfer to a slow cooker. Set on low heat and allow to work until dumplings begin to fall apart, about 2 hours. Change to the warm setting to avoid burning. Serve with cheddar cheese.

Chef Tips
The key that made my mom go back for seconds and thirds was adding the red wine vinegar to remove the weight from the dish.

There are two forms of chicken and dumplings. The thin version that is similar to chicken noodle soup and the heavier cream sauce version that I have here.

I had been experimenting on many different foods, ingredients, and cooking methods before I got to this recipe. When I made this recipe for the first time while applying all of the theories that are now contained within this book, it was the first time in weeks that my mom was able to come up with an appetite of any kind for a meal. You cannot imagine my relief in watching my mom go back for seconds and even thirds! This is where it all came together into a complete understanding of everything that she was experiencing. As a result, this is the recipe from whence *Cooking for Chemo* was born.

CHICKEN GUMBO

Recipe Description

The classic creole dish featuring the obligatory "holy trinity" of peppers, onions, and celery. The holy trinity is the Cajun version of mirepoix. Gumbo is fantastic in that it is both light and flavorful at the same time.

Tasting Guidelines

Taste is savory, a little spicy, and aromatic.
Weight is light, but can be balanced with vinegar and tomatoes.
Texture is soupy.
Good for people with low to moderate treatment side effects.
Emotional response of good ole' Cajun love.
Best categorized as Cajun.

Ingredients

2 lbs. chicken breast, cut into ½" chunks
1 c. rice, cooked
1 large can tomatoes
2 green peppers, cored, diced, seeded
1 yellow onion, diced
4 celery stalks, chopped
1 bag okra, frozen
2 large cans chicken broth
oil/butter

Flavor Balancers

kosher salt to taste
black pepper to taste
cayenne pepper
red wine vinegar

Aromatics

2 tbsp. garlic, minced
2 bay leaves

Recipe Directions

Bring a large pot to a medium heat. Add 1 to 2 tbsp. of oil or butter for sautéing. Sauté onions, green peppers, celery, and garlic. Cook until translucent. At this point, stir in chicken breast, cut into ½" chunks. Sauté chicken until lightly brown and cooked thoroughly. Salt and pepper. After the chicken is done, lightly deglaze the pan with red wine vinegar. Allow to reduce. Stir in tomatoes, chicken broth, and par cooked rice. Bring to a boil. Cook until rice is finished. When rice is finished, reduce to a medium heat. Stir in okra. Taste and adjust seasonings as needed. Allow to simmer 10 minutes until okra is thoroughly cooked. Serve immediately.

Chef Tips

This recipe employs what is referred to in Cajun and creole food as "the holy trinity." The holy trinity is onions, celery, and green peppers. This forms the base for that traditional Louisiana flavor. Also, see cornbread recipe in the snacks section. It goes well with this recipe.

Be careful with the rice. As a little can go a long way. If you put in too much rice, you will end up with a rice dish (not a soup) that tastes like gumbo. I have learned this from experience.

CHICKEN NOODLE SOUP

Recipe Description

An American classic. If there is somebody in the United States that has never heard of chicken noodle soup, they must live under the world's largest rock. This dish is what I consider to be a slightly up-market take on the dish. This chicken noodle soup features big cuts of veggies, egg noodles, and a good aromatic quality.

Tasting Guidelines

Taste is savory and aromatic.

Weight is light, but can be balanced with sugar and red wine vinegar.

Texture is soupy.

Good for people with moderate to severe treatment side effects.

Emotional response of being loved when you are sick.

Best categorized as classic American.

Ingredients

½ lb. chicken breast, cooked and chopped
1-24 oz. pack of egg noodles, cooked
½ c. onion, chopped
½ c. celery, chopped
½ c. carrots, sliced
2 large can chicken broth
1 tbsp. oil

Flavor Balancers

kosher salt to taste
1 tsp. light soy sauce or ½ tbsp. MSG
black pepper to taste
1 tbsp. red wine vinegar
1 tbsp. sugar

Aromatics

2 bay leaves
1 tbsp. ground sage

Recipe Directions

Heat oil and 1 c. water in a large spaghetti pot over medium heat. Cook the onion, celery, and carrots until tender allowing the water to reduce, sautéing the vegetables after the water evaporates. Add chicken and sauté lightly as well. Add seasonings and broth. Allow to come to a boil. Reduce from a boil and allow to simmer 30 minutes. Add egg noodles 5 minutes before serving. Remove bay leaves immediately before serving.

Chef Tips

For a more savory soup, add a small can of diced tomatoes, mushrooms, 1 tbsp. dark soy sauce, or 1 tbsp. MSG. For a little kick, add a little cayenne pepper in the beginning of cooking. It will help with any congestion in the head. A little red wine vinegar can help ease a queasy stomach as can a few slices of peeled fresh ginger and soy sauce. Do not eat the slices of ginger. Remove before serving.

CHILI

Texas Disclaimer
To all the Texans out there,
Yes! I realize that "real" chili has no beans in it. But, the purpose of this recipe is to provide a friendly,
well-rounded chili that everyone can enjoy.

Recipe Description
This is a family recipe passed down from my grandfather to me. I have slightly modified it to make
it friendlier for chemo and lighter over all. It is a good, all-around chili. It is very versatile and can be
eaten as a meal, over pasta, or even over hot dogs if you like.

Tasting Guidelines
Taste is savory, peppery, and a little sweet and tangy.
Weight is medium, but can be balanced with vinegar and ketchup.
Texture is soft and chili like.
Good for people with low to moderate treatment side effects.
Emotional response of feeling warm on a cold winters night.
Best categorized as classic American.

Ingredients
1 lb. lean *(at least 90/10 or leaner)* ground beef
2 large cans of chili beans
or red kidney beans, undrained
1 large can tomatoes, diced and undrained
2 green peppers, cored and medium diced
1 large onion, medium diced
1 tbsp. oil

Flavor Balancers
3 tsp. kosher salt
2 tbsp. soy sauce
½ tbsp. cayenne pepper
2 tbsp. red wine vinegar
2 tbsp. sugar

Aromatics
2 tbsp. garlic, minced
1 tbsp. cumin, ground
2 tbsp. dried oregano
2 tbsp. chili powder *(optional)*

Recipe Directions
In a large sauté pan or skillet, bring oil to medium heat. Add garlic, onions, and green pepper.
Lightly sauté for 5 minutes. Add enough water to lightly cover the ingredients. Cover pan and allow
to sweat until onions are translucent.

Break up ground beef. Add to sauté pan, mixing all ingredients together. Cook beef thoroughly and
try to keep the ground beef chunks as small as possible. Now you will add the diced tomatoes, black
pepper, salt, cumin, chili powder, cayenne pepper, and soy sauce. Cover with water, and allow to
simmer and reduce. Similar to how you make homemade tacos.

Reduce liquid until it forms a bit of sauce at the very bottom. If your sauté pan is large enough, add remaining ingredients, stirring thoroughly and allowing to simmer on low heat for a couple hours. If pan is not big enough, transfer to spaghetti pot and repeat above method. For ease and convenience, I like my chili to simmer in a slow cooker so I don't burn it.

The idea here is the longer the flavors sit together, the better they taste. Serve with your favorite chili condiments, like oyster crackers, sour dough bread bowl, freshly chopped onions, cheddar cheese, hot sauce, etc. Whatever you like or whatever your chemo patient is able to eat.

Chef Tips
If chili is heavy, add red wine vinegar and sugar to lighten the flavor. A little rice really adds some substance to this chili recipe! Feel free to experiment! If you feel like your chili might be missing something, I highly recommend adding some ketchup.

CLAM CHOWDER

Recipe Description
Clam chowder is one of my personal favorites. This is a classic New England style recipe, and not to be confused with the tomato-based Manhattan clam chowder. The key to a good clam chowder is getting good clams. If you can't get good clams, you might as well make baked potato soup.

Tasting Guidelines
Taste is savory and a little salty.
Weight is heavy, but can be balanced with lemon juice and sugar.
Texture is that of a thickened soup.
Good for people with low treatment side effects.
Emotional response of a warm hearty fisherman's dish.
Best categorized as classic American.

Ingredients
1 large can chicken broth
2-10 oz. cans clams, chopped, in juice
(reduce to one can if nose is very sensitive)
1 lb. red potatoes, cut into thumb nail size cubes,
(optional)
3 carrots, medium diced
3 celery stalks, medium diced
1 yellow onion, medium diced
4 slices crispy bacon, chopped,
(optional, but recommended)
¼ c. green onions, thinly sliced
1 stick butter
½ c. flour
1 c. heavy whipping cream

Flavor Balancers
½ tbsp. freshly ground black pepper
1 tsp. cayenne pepper
1 tsp. white pepper
2 tbsp. lemon juice

Aromatics
1-2 tbsp. Old Bay seasoning

Recipe Directions
Melt butter in a large spaghetti pot over medium heat. Add in onions, celery, and carrots. Cook until onions are translucent. Stir in flour until butter is absorbed thoroughly. Add chicken stock, and bring to a high heat. Add potatoes and boil until tender. Add seasonings a little bit at a time adjusting as you go. Pour in clam juice only. Add cream. Reduce over medium heat. Taste again for flavors, adding more seasonings if necessary. Add clams, bacon, green onion, and lemon juice 10 minutes before serving and reduce to a low heat.

Chef Tips
I personally like my clam chowder to be visually appealing, which is why I add carrots, bacon, and green onions to mine. The reason you always want to add seafood in the last 10 minutes of cooking

is so you don't overcook the seafood. When clams are over-cooked, they become rubbery, which nobody likes. If you are concerned about texture, but want to keep the clam chowder flavor, use the juice of two cans of clams and omit the clams physically. I also personally recommend chopping the clams into smaller pieces so that their texture becomes more integrated into the dish.

COCONUT CURRY STEW

Recipe Description
One of my personal favorite Asian soups. Whether it is specifically Vietnamese or Thai, is something for somebody else to debate. All I care is that it is freaking delicious!

Tasting Guidelines
Taste is sweet and spicy with aromatic curry notes.
Weight is medium, but can be balanced with lemon grass.
Texture is soupy.
Good for people with low to moderate treatment side effects.
Emotional response of unexpected goodness.
Best categorized as Southeast Asian.

Ingredients
3 chicken breast
3 red potatoes, chunked
1 small bag of carrots, chunked
1 onion red yellow or white
½ celery bunch, chopped
1 can coconut milk
2 c. cow's milk
32 oz. chicken stock/broth *(low sodium)*

Flavor Balancers
kosher salt to taste
black pepper to taste

Aromatics
1 tsp. ground ginger
2 tsp. cinnamon
1 tbsp. lemon grass, pureed
2 bay leaves
3 tbsp. red curry

Recipe Directions
Chunk up all vegetables and meat. Place all ingredients, flavor balancers, and aromatics in slow cooker on high for 4 hours. Add salt and pepper to taste. Serve with jasmine rice on side.

Chef Tips
Lemon grass adds a nice, clean finish, especially for people who are having trouble with flavors. This curry should be sweet. Add sugar as needed, especially to combat metallic tastes. For metallic tastes, add ½ a lime sliced into cocktail wedges with juice. Remove limes before serving.

CRAB AND LOBSTER BISQUE

Recipe Description

This recipe is one of my personal favorites. Call me decadent, but I like to personally use crab and lobster. The weight of this dish is much lighter than it seems when done correctly. This dish is also very easy to make. As a rule of thumb, bisque is always lighter in weight than chowder.

Tasting Guidelines

Taste is savory and aromatic.
Weight is medium, but can be balanced with lemon juice.
Texture is a thickened soup.
Good for people with low to moderate treatment side effects.
Emotional response of a delicious high end quality dinner.
Best categorized as French.

Ingredients

1 pack imitation crab meat, chunk or flake style, it does not matter
1 pack imitation lobster meat, chunk or flake style, it does not matter
1 small box portabella mushrooms, finely chopped
1 large yellow onion
1 family-sized can cream mushroom soup
1 family-sized can tomato soup or tomato bisque
whole milk
2 sticks butter
flour for roux

Flavor Balancers

1 tsp. salt
½ tbsp. black pepper
1 tsp. cayenne pepper
2 tbsp. red wine vinegar
juice of one lemon

Aromatics

2 tbsp. garlic, minced
2 bay leaves
2 tbsp. Old Bay seasoning

Recipe Directions

In a large spaghetti pot, melt butter over medium heat. Sauté onions, mushrooms, and garlic together allowing mushrooms to really release their juices. Cover and allow to simmer over low heat if necessary. Low heat will help prevent the garlic from burning.

Next, take half of the lobster and crab meat and put it into the pot. Add seasonings and stir thoroughly so every inch is coated. Bring pan to a medium heat and use a smashing or chopping technique to break down the crab and lobster into a sort of puree. Add lemon juice.

Next, stir in flour to absorb the extra butter. Then add the canned soups. Fill cans full of milk and add to pot, stirring over a medium-low heat until everything is mixed thoroughly. Allow to warm, stirring frequently and ensuring the soup does not burn.

At this point, it is important to take note of the flavors as they will change throughout cooking. Because of the canned tomato soup not being properly cooked all the way, you will notice a tangy almost ketchup-like flavor at this point. You will know when the soup is ready to be served because the flavor will stop being tangy and will instead become very rich and savory. At this point, add your remaining lobster and crab. Allow to warm for 10 minutes and enjoy.

Chef Tips
You can definitely use fresh or canned meat in substitute of the imitation meat. I personally prefer it. But with a can of blue crab going for fifteen dollars plus currently, I tend not to use it. The longer this soup cooks the better it tastes! This is also a fantastic slow cooker dish. Perform the above steps on the stove until the point of mixing in the canned soups and instead combine in a slow cooker. Allow to work overnight on low or for 4 hours on high. The slow cooker is a fantastic way to avoid burning the soup.

CUCUMBER AND YOGURT SOUP (CHILLED)

Recipe Description
A very light and refreshing dish. Perfect for hot summer days or when you are just feeling classy enough to have a chilled soup. This dish is very good for those who have a strong metallic taste.

Tasting Guidelines
Taste is tangy and fresh.
Weight is light, but can be balanced with sugar.
Texture is a cream soup.
Good for people with low to severe treatment side effects.
Emotional response of I'm so fancy.
Best categorized as Mediterranean.

Ingredients
3 c. honey Greek yogurt
1 large cucumber, peeled and shredded
3 tbsp. extra virgin olive oil
1 c. cold water

Flavor Balancers
kosher salt to taste
freshly ground black pepper to taste
1 tbsp. red wine vinaigrette

Aromatics
1 tbsp. garlic, minced
1 tbsp. fresh dill, finely chopped
2 tbsp. fresh mint, finely chopped

Recipe Directions
Shred cucumbers with a cheese grater into a large colander. Lightly toss cucumbers with kosher salt. Allow to sit in sink about 20 minutes. This allows time to draw out the extra moisture from the cucumbers.

In a large bowl, mix remaining ingredients *(except water)*. Taste for saltiness. Adjust seasonings if necessary. Slowly, mix in cold water until a thin and soupy texture is created.

At this point, all the ingredients should have very distinct flavors, and the dish should be light, creamy, and refreshing. Allow to refrigerate at least 4 hours for flavors to work together. Serve chilled.

Chef Tips
Serve with fresh pitas or crusty bread. Like Tzatziki, this soup can be served as a dip, garnish, or sauce by omitting the water.

FRENCH ONION SOUP

Recipe Description
French onion soup is a classic French recipe loved the world over. Rich savory beef broth, caramelized onions, crunchy croutons, and melty Swiss cheese create a symphony of decadent flavors. In France, onion soup is used as a hangover cure after a long night of wine drinking.

Tasting Guidelines
Taste is savory.
Weight is medium.
Texture is soft.
Good for people with low to moderate side effects.
Emotional response of warm, well-loved goodness.
Best categorized as classic French.

Ingredients
3 qt. beef stock
1 bottle Cabernet Sauvignon
3 lbs. yellow onions, sliced into thin strips
1 baguette, sliced into ½" thick circles
1 lb. Swiss cheese, grated
1 stick of butter *(¼ c., 4 oz.)*

Flavor Balancers
2 tsp. kosher salt
½ tbsp. black pepper
1 tsp. red wine vinegar
1 tbsp. sugar

Aromatics
2 bay leaves

Recipe Directions
Soup
Heat a large spaghetti pot with a lid over medium heat. Melt your butter. Add onions, pepper, and kosher salt. Toss onions and butter together until completely mixed. Cover with lid and allow to cook 15 minutes. Toss the onions and butter together again until the bottom onions are now the top onions. Repeat these steps until onions are thoroughly soft and caramelized. When onions are translucent, begin adding wine a few ounces at a time. Mix the onions and the wine together and allow the wine to almost cook completely out before adding more wine. Repeat this process until the entire bottle of wine has been added and reduced. Repeat this process again with one quart of beef stock. Take care to not allow beef stock or wine to burn as this will carry a smoky smell through the

entire soup.

After wine and beef stock have been reduced, add remaining beef stock, sugar, red wine, and bay leaf. Allow to simmer 30 minutes for optimum flavor. Onion soup should be very rich and savory. Look for a touch of sweetness with the addition of sugar. Not noticeably sweet, but a touch sweet for balance.

Croutons
Preheat your oven to 375°F. Place baguette slices on baking sheet. Place sheet into oven and allow slices to dry out until they are almost completely brown all over. The purpose of this is to dry the bread out as much as possible. Dry bread soaks up more soup and makes for a much more delicious experience.

Serving
Ladle soup into a bowl, filling no more than ⅔ of the bowl with soup. Place a generous amount of croutons on top of the soup. Cover croutons with a handful of grated Swiss cheese. Either microwave for 30 seconds, or place under broiler to melt cheese.

Chef Tips
The key to this soup is the slow cooking of the onions and the slow addition and reduction of the wine and beef stock. This process is called "au sec." This process reduces the water content and condenses the concentration of flavor. When you reduce the wine and stock, the end product should look like melted chocolate or fudge.

GAZPACHO (COLD)

Recipe Description
Gazpacho is probably the most iconic Spanish dish that I can think of. It is also great for people with severe treatment side effects as its construction makes it naturally light and refreshing.

Tasting Guidelines
Taste is savory and light.
Weight is light, but can be balanced with vinegar.
Texture is soupy.
Good for people with low to severe treatment side effects.
Especially metallic tastes.
Emotional response of summer time freshness.
Best categorized as classic Spanish.

Ingredients
1 large can tomatoes, diced
3 ripe Roma tomatoes, cored and chunked into small ½" chunks
2 medium-sized green bell peppers, medium diced
1 green cucumber, medium diced
1 medium red onion, medium diced
olive oil

Flavor Balancers
kosher salt to taste
1 tsp. Worcestershire sauce
black pepper to taste
¼ tsp. cayenne pepper
red wine vinaigrette dressing
juice of 1 lime
¼ c. sugar

Aromatics
2 tbsp. garlic, minced
½ tsp. ground cumin
fresh basil, thinly sliced for garnish

Recipe Directions
In a large sauté pan, bring 1 tbsp. of olive oil to a medium heat. Sauté garlic, 1 green pepper, and ½ of the red onion until the onion is cooked. Add diced tomatoes and cayenne pepper, simmering over medium heat 45 minutes. While cooking, break down tomatoes, green peppers, and red onion with a whisk by smashing and whisking vigorously to puree sauce. Add sugar and a splash of red wine vinaigrette dressing when tomatoes have sufficiently broken down. Season with pepper and salt to taste.

Transfer into a large mixing bowl and allow to chill overnight. In a separate bowl, combine remaining ingredients (except basil) and marinate with red wine vinaigrette dressing overnight. The next morning combine everything into one bowl. Garnish with fresh basil for a cleansing pop. Serve chilled with crusty bread or croutons.

GREEK LENTIL SOUP

Recipe Description

Lentil soup is a classic all across the Mediterranean. But, this recipe is from the island of Cypress. Very filling while still being light. This dish is packed full of vitamins, minerals, protein, and flavor.

Tasting Guidelines

Taste is savory and spicy.

Weight is light, but can be balanced with sugar.

Texture is soft.

Good for people with low to moderate treatment side effects.

Emotional response of a nice healthy meal.

Best categorized as classic Greek.

Ingredients

1 lb. green lentils, washed
1 red onion, medium diced
1 large can tomatoes, diced
4 carrots, thinly sliced
4 celery stalks, thinly sliced
2 green peppers, medium diced

Flavor Balancers

2 tbsp. soy sauce
2 tsp. cayenne pepper
3 tbsp. red wine vinegar
¼ c. sugar

Aromatics

2 heaping tbsp. garlic, minced
2 large bay leaves
1 tsp. cumin, ground
1 tbsp. red curry powder

Recipe Directions

In a large slow cooker, combine all ingredients. Leave room to add water. Add water so it covers ingredients an extra 1" in depth. Allow to cook on high 6-8 hours, stirring occasionally making sure lentils don't stick to the bottom. The longer you cook this dish, the less grainy the lentils will be.

This dish holds on warm in the slow cooker very well. If soup becomes too thick, or gets a bit of a film on it, simply stir in more water to remedy. Lentils drink water when cooking. If soup is too thin, and you desire a little thickness to the soup, mix in a little properly prepared cornstarch.

Chef Tips

This can be portioned and refrigerated or frozen. This dish is extremely high in protein and dietary fiber. If you can just get one soup ladle into someone, it will really pack a wallop.

HOT AND SOUR SOUP

Recipe Description
The Chinese restaurant classic! Spicy, savory, and a little sour. It is most definitely an acquired taste. But once you develop your palate for this soup, you will find yourself craving it on cold winter days!

Tasting Guidelines
Taste is spicy, savory, and sour.
Weight is medium.
Texture is soft and soupy.
Good for people with low to severe treatment side effects.
Emotional response of spicy, tangy, metallic taste relief.
Best categorized as Chinese American.

Ingredients
4 oz. firm tofu, sliced into ¼" x ¼" x1" strips
⅔ c. wood ear mushrooms, chopped fine
½ c. bamboo shoots, thin julienne
½ c. carrots, thin julienne
2 tbsp. cornstarch with 2 tbsp. water *(cornstarch slurry)*
3 eggs, scrambled smooth, uncooked
3 qt. hot water

Flavor Balancers
½ c. soy sauce
¼ c. rice vinegar
¼ c. sugar
½ tbsp. black pepper, ground
1 tsp. black pepper, ground
2 Chinese red peppers
½ tbsp. white pepper, ground

Recipe Directions
In a large spaghetti pot, bring water to a boil. Add all flavor balancers and return to a boil. Add mushrooms, bamboo shoots, and carrots. Return to a boil, and allow to boil together about 30 minutes. Taste soup for flavor. Soup should be savory, spicy, and sour with a touch of sweetness to mellow the soup. If flavor is correct, stir in the cornstarch slurry, and return to a boil for 5 min to thicken the soup. Reduce heat to medium-low and slowly stir in tofu, cover with a lid and allow to simmer 15 additional minutes. Remove pot from heat. Put eggs into a liquid measuring cup with a pour spout. Slowly pour scrambled eggs into broth. The key is to create thin long ribbons of eggs. This is achieved by pouring the eggs out slowly in a long ribbon-like motion. Start at one end of the pot, begin to slowly pour and move your hand to the other side of the pot. Then stop pouring at

the other end. Use a fork or preferably, chop sticks to slowly move ribbons of egg through the soup. Do not whisk. Do not return to a boil. Repeat this motion allowing the egg to cook for about 30 seconds in-between ribbons. After egg has been added and cooked, give it a good stir and it is ready to serve!

Chef Tips
Using exact proportions of sugar and vinegar allows the soup to be sour, but balanced. If the soup isn't sour enough add extra vinegar to add that refreshing sour pop.
If wood ear mushrooms are unavailable in your area, baby bella *(crimini)* mushrooms are an effective and flavorful substitution.

Wood ear mushrooms have a unique flavor and texture. Uncooked they are not very aromatic or flavorful with a texture akin to rubber. But when you cook them down, they develop a rich almost beefy flavor and a jelly-like texture. This is why I recommend chopping them as finely as possible, they release more flavor this way and there is no strange texture to notice!

MATZO BALL SOUP

Recipe Description
A Jewish classic! Matzo Ball Soup is the Jewish equivalent of Chicken Noodle Soup, with the biggest variation being dumplings made from matzo meal instead of pasta. This is a very filling and delicious soup full of warm flavors that will make you feel loved.

Tasting Guidelines
Taste is salty and savory.
Weight is light.
Texture is soft.
Good for low to severe side effects.
Emotional response of feeling like a kid again.
Best categorized as Jewish comfort food.

Ingredients
1 c. matzo meal
2 eggs, uncooked and scrambled
½ c. water
1 chicken breast, roughly chopped
3 celery stalks, thinly sliced
1 yellow onion, thinly sliced
3 carrots thinly, sliced
3 qt. chicken broth
2 tbsp. olive oil

Flavor Balancers
kosher salt to taste
black pepper to taste
1 tsp. red wine vinegar
1 tsp. sugar

Aromatics
2 tsp. rubbed sage
2 tsp. old bay seasoning
2 bay leaves

Recipe Directions
Matzo Balls
In a medium mixing bowl, add matzo, eggs, water, and 1 tsp. salt. Mix together until all water is absorbed and matzo forms a firm paste. Allow mixture to rest approximately 20 minutes.

Soup
Heat a large spaghetti pot over medium heat. Add olive oil, celery, onion, chicken, and carrots. Stir fry until onions are translucent and chicken is thoroughly cooked. Add red wine vinegar to deglaze pan. Add aromatics, seasonings, and chicken broth. Bring soup to a boil.

After soup boils for 10 minutes, remove matzo paste from refrigerator. Grab a small glass and fill with water. Wet your fingers with water and use a small teaspoon to form 1" or smaller balls out of the matzo mix. After forming the balls drop them into the boiling soup. When all balls have been made, cover the pot, and reduce to a medium simmer. Allow matzo balls to simmer at least 40 minutes. After matzo balls are fully cooked, serve.

Chef Tips
The longer the soup simmers with the matzo balls, the better the matzo balls will taste, as they absorb the soup broth.

MINESTRONE WITH PESTO

Recipe Description
A classic take on minestrone soup. The pesto really sets off the freshness of the dish. If you have a nut allergy, omit the pine nuts from the pesto. This soup really puts the emphasis on the old joke that soup is made out of leftovers and throw away parts.

Tasting Guidelines
Taste is light, but savory.
Weight is light, but can be balanced with tomatoes and sugar.
Texture is soupy.
Good for people with low to severe treatment side effects.
Emotional response of eating a home cooked Italian meal.
Best categorized as classic Italian.

Ingredients
1 small can cannellini beans or great northern beans
1 box of tri-color rotini noodles, cooked
2 yellow onions, chopped
2 carrots, diced
2 celery stalks, chopped
3 red potatoes, diced
1 large can tomatoes, diced
4 oz. green beans, cut in short lengths
2 zucchini, diced
¼ c. olive oil
8 c. water

Flavor Balancers
kosher salt to taste
freshly ground black pepper to taste
2 tbsp. red wine vinegar
1 tbsp. sugar

Aromatics
2 tbsp. garlic, minced
4 tbsp. pesto sauce

Recipe Directions
In a large spaghetti pot, bring oil to a medium heat. Sauté garlic, carrots, onion, and celery until onions are translucent but garlic is not burned. Add remaining ingredients except for pasta. Boil until potatoes are tender. Add cooked pasta 10 minutes before serving and reduce to a low heat.

MULLIGATAWNY SOUP

Recipe Description
A classic Indian soup. A perfect soup for hot days. The apples in this dish really lighten it up and leave you feeling refreshed.

Tasting Guidelines
Taste is light and sweet.
Weight is light, but can be balanced with sugar.
Texture is soupy.
Good for people with low to severe treatment side effects.
Best categorized as classic Europeanized Indian.

Ingredients
1 c. chicken, cooked and diced
1 c. white rice, cooked
2 granny smith apples, peeled, cored and diced
1 c. onions, diced
4 to 6 carrots, diced
4 celery stalks, diced
8 c. chicken stock
1 c. cream, hot
½ c. butter
3 tbsp. cornstarch, mixed into 1 c. cold water

Flavor Balancers
2 tsp. kosher salt
½ tsp. freshly ground black pepper

Aromatics
1 tsp. ground ginger
4 tsp. red curry powder
1 tsp. dried thyme

Recipe Directions
Bring a large spaghetti pot to a medium heat. Melt the butter. After melting the butter, sauté the onions, carrots, and celery. Add chicken and seasonings. Mix thoroughly. Add chicken stock. Bring to a boil. Add rice and cream. Mix thoroughly. Taste the soup and adjust flavors as needed.

The next thing you want to do is add the cornstarch and apples. At this point, we want to taste the soup again. The soup should be light, warm, and crisp. If it's not light, warm, and crisp with a touch of sweetness, add a little vinegar and a little sugar.

Chef Tips
This soup is really good as a light, but flavorful meal. It is perfect for somebody who is having trouble keeping down heavier foods. The ginger, cream, and rice will have a calming effect on their stomach. For someone with mouth sores, omit red curry and use yellow curry.

PEACH AND YOGURT SOUP

Recipe Description
A delicious treat for when you are not feeling so hot. This is a sweet and entertaining dish that is perfect for days when you are not feeling very good and need a little pick-me-up in spirit. This dish is just great for when you are down in the dumps.

Tasting Guidelines
Taste is creamy and sweet.
Weight is light, but can be balanced with peach schnapps and white wine.
Texture is creamy.
Good for people with low to severe treatment side effects.
Emotional response of a delicious treat on a hot summer day.
Best categorized as cold soup.

Ingredients
8 oz. Greek yogurt
10 fresh peach slices
2 c. half-and-half cream
1 c. peach schnapps

Flavor Balancers
1 c. sweet white wine
½ c. sugar

Aromatics
½ tsp. cinnamon, ground
¼ tsp. nutmeg, ground
1 tsp. fresh mint leaves, chopped

Recipe Directions
Combine all ingredients in a large spaghetti pot. Cook over a medium heat until peaches are tender being careful not to scorch the cream. Remove from heat when peaches are nice and tender. Cool down soup and blend in a blender or mash peaches with a whisk. Cover and refrigerate until ready to serve. Serve chilled.

Chef Tips
For a more homemade look, do not mash the peaches but cut them into small pieces. Also note that as soon as the dish hits proper temperature, the alcohol from the wine and the schnapps will evaporate leaving its flavor but not its intoxicating effects. This renders it safe for all ages.

POTATO LEEK SOUP (COLD)

Recipe Description
Never underestimate the power of a cold soup. Chilled soups are great for hot days, adding variety to a meal, and especially good for people who have very severe mouth sores. Sometimes mouth sores can get so bad that hot soup can burn in your mouth. This soup is a good alternative to feeling that kind of mouth pain. It is a great way to return hope to somebody who has lost it. French accent when serving is optional.

Tasting Guidelines
Taste is savory.
Weight is medium, but can be balanced with red wine vinegar.
Texture is soupy and cold.
Good for people with low to severe treatment side effects.
Emotional response of a fancy French dish.
Best categorized as French.

Ingredients
1 lb. leeks, chopped into small pieces with dark green sections removed
3 yellow potatoes, peeled and diced small
1 tbsp. chives, thinly sliced
1 large can vegetable broth
½ stick unsalted butter
1 c. heavy cream
1 c. buttermilk

Flavor Balancers
kosher salt to taste
1 tsp. white pepper

Recipe Directions
In a large spaghetti pot over medium heat, melt the butter. Add the leeks with 1 tsp. of kosher salt. Sweat for 30 minutes covered, stirring occasionally. When leeks are tender, add potatoes and vegetable broth. Bring pot to a boil over medium-high heat until potatoes are tender about 30-45 minutes. Using a whisk, whisk the potatoes and leeks until they are thoroughly mashed and blended together. Remove from heat, and add remaining ingredients. Season until desired taste is reached. Serve either chilled or warm.

WONTON SOUP

Recipe Description
A Chinese restaurant classic. The warm ginger and hearty pork dumplings make this delicious soup a classic comfort food.

Tasting Guidelines
Taste is savory.
Weight is light.
Texture is soft and soupy.
Good for people with low to severe treatment side effects.
Emotional response of love and comfort.
Best categorized as Chinese American.

Ingredients
1 lb. fresh ground pork
1 green onion, sliced thin
1 egg
2 tsp. bread crumbs
4 qt. chicken stock
2 oz. fresh wood ear mushrooms or portabella mushrooms, chopped fine
1 pack wonton wrappers

Flavor Balancers
1 tsp. dark soy sauce
2 tbsp. light soy sauce
1 tsp. black pepper, ground

Aromatics
2 tbsp. garlic, minced
2 tbsp. ginger. peeled and minced

Garnish
1 green onion, sliced thin

Recipe Directions
Wonton Filling
Add garlic, mushrooms, ginger and green onions to a food processor and process until extremely fine and almost paste-like. In a large bowl add ground pork, mushrooms, garlic, ginger, green onions, egg, bread crumbs, dark soy sauce, light soy sauce, and black pepper. Mix all ingredients together until mixture is smooth and looks like meatball or hamburger mixture. Allow flavors to marinade together at least 30 minutes. Overnight is even better.

Making the Dumplings

Making dumplings is much easier as a two person operation. One to fill the dumplings, and one to seal the dumplings. Using a large baking sheet, lay out wonton skins so that the dumplings may be made quickly. Fill a small cup with water and place to side of baking sheet. Using your thumb and forefinger, place approximately 1 tsp. of filling into the center of each dumpling. After all wonton skins have filling, wash your hands of the filling mixture and begin to seal the dumplings. Use water from the cup we placed out earlier to line the edges with water and then fold them into triangular packages. Make certain that there are no air bubbles in the dumplings. Repeat this set of actions until all dumplings have been made. Keep in mind that extra dumplings can be packaged and frozen for later use.

Cooking the Dumplings and Serving the Soup

Bring the chicken broth to a boil and then lower the heat to a low simmer. Place as many dumplings as you can eat into the broth and allow to simmer, stirring occasionally for about 20-30 minutes or until the dumpling filling is fully cooked. Place dumplings and broth into a bowl. Garnish with a few slices of green onion and serve.

Chef Tips

For a more authentic flavor, finish with a drop or two of sesame oil. I like to cook a little ginger into the broth for a warmer soup flavor. Wonton soup is extremely versatile. I make a wonton noodle soup version at home. This is where I cut the wontons into thin noodles, and use the dumpling filling as meatballs in the soup.

Recipe Name	Date and Time Eaten	Rating

Recipe Source	Est. Calories

Ingredients and Seasonings

Describe the Taste?

What did you Like?

What did you NOT Like?

What can you add or subtract?

Describe the Texture	Describe the Smell
Any Complications?	How did this recipe make you feel?

Additional Tasting Notes

Recipe Name	Date and Time Eaten	Rating

Recipe Source	Est. Calories

Ingredients and Seasonings

Describe the Taste?

What did you Like?

What did you NOT Like?

What can you add or subtract?

Describe the Texture	Describe the Smell
Any Complications?	How did this recipe make you feel?

Additional Tasting Notes

Recipe Name	Date and Time Eaten	Rating
Recipe Source		Est. Calories

Ingredients and Seasonings

Describe the Taste?

What did you Like?

What did you NOT Like?

What can you add or subtract?

Describe the Texture	Describe the Smell
Any Complications?	How did this recipe make you feel?

Additional Tasting Notes

Recipe Name	Date and Time Eaten	Rating

Recipe Source	Est. Calories

Ingredients and Seasonings

Describe the Taste?

What did you Like?

What did you NOT Like?

What can you add or subtract?

Describe the Texture	Describe the Smell

Any Complications?	How did this recipe make you feel?

Additional Tasting Notes

Recipe Name	Date and Time Eaten	Rating
Recipe Source		Est. Calories

Ingredients and Seasonings

Describe the Taste?

What did you Like?

What did you NOT Like?

What can you add or subtract?

Describe the Texture	Describe the Smell
Any Complications?	How did this recipe make you feel?

Additional Tasting Notes

Recipe Name	Date and Time Eaten	Rating
Recipe Source		Est. Calories

Ingredients and Seasonings

Describe the Taste?

What did you Like?

What did you NOT Like?

What can you add or subtract?

Describe the Texture	Describe the Smell
Any Complications?	How did this recipe make you feel?

Additional Tasting Notes

Recipe Name	Date and Time Eaten	Rating

Recipe Source	Est. Calories

Ingredients and Seasonings

Describe the Taste?

What did you Like?

What did you NOT Like?

What can you add or subtract?

Describe the Texture	Describe the Smell
Any Complications?	How did this recipe make you feel?

Additional Tasting Notes

Recipe Name	Date and Time Eaten	Rating
Recipe Source		Est. Calories

Ingredients and Seasonings

Describe the Taste?

What did you Like?

What did you NOT Like?

What can you add or subtract?

Describe the Texture	Describe the Smell
Any Complications?	How did this recipe make you feel?

Additional Tasting Notes

Recipe Name	Date and Time Eaten	Rating

Recipe Source	Est. Calories

Ingredients and Seasonings

Describe the Taste?

What did you Like?

What did you NOT Like?

What can you add or subtract?

Describe the Texture	Describe the Smell
Any Complications?	How did this recipe make you feel?

Additional Tasting Notes

SMOOTHIE RECIPES

Smoothies are amazing! The flavor combinations are literally endless. They are also great for sneaking super healthy things into your body without you even noticing. What I love about smoothies is that they can be a simple and flavorful treat or they can act as an entire meal replacement. Smoothies are great as snacks or as a substitute for a heavy meal when you have severe mouth sores.

The way I think about smoothies is the way I think about ice cream. Whatever flavor combinations of ice cream you like are naturally going to be the flavors of smoothies you like. For example, I personally love chocolate ice cream! As a result, one of my favorite smoothie flavor combinations is chocolate, strawberry, and banana. Think about the results of your tasting experiments, what flavors did you like? What flavors did your loved one have the most success with? Use these flavors as a starting point to craft smoothies that will be both delicious and edible.

In the following section, we will give you a handful of flavorful recipes and how to prepare them.

Prepping and Storing Ingredients

If you are pressed for time, you can always prep your smoothie meal ahead of time so when you are hungry you can just blend and drink.

There are many ways to make your life easier. One easy way is simply portioning the ingredients into food storage bags and either refrigerating or freezing them. You can portion them for an entire day or even for the week.

For yogurt, you can simply take an ice cube try, fill it with yogurt, and freeze it. After the yogurt is frozen, you can add the yogurt cubes to your pre-portioned freezer bags. If that is too much extra work, you can always just add the yogurt to the blender when you are ready to make the smoothie.

For storage of ingredients, you always want to make sure everything is properly prepared and sealed to prevent any cross-contamination or food poisoning. I used mostly frozen fruits for my mom while she was going through chemo. Because there is no safe way to decontaminate fresh fruits and vegetables, using frozen fruits and vegetables lowers the risk of accidentally getting food poisoning. If you have any further questions, feel free to reference the *Food Safety and Sanitation* lesson.

Palate Cleansing with Smoothies

To properly do a palate cleanse to remove that nasty metallic taste from someone's mouth, instead of using vinegar like we would use in a cooked dish, we want to use citrus juices in smoothies instead. Examples of this would be lemons, limes, and oranges. The citric acid cuts through the metallic taste. Its acidity helps to leave a clean feeling in your mouth. A great example of a smoothie that palate cleanses very well is our blueberry lemon smoothie. Other acidic and tart flavors, like green apples, work as well.

General Smoothie Directions

Preparing smoothies is very easy and simple.

1. Add all ingredients into the blender and cover.

2. Activate the blender. If you have frozen ingredients that refuse to be chopped, use the pulse function and a little finesse to pulse your way into the perfect mixture.

3. Taste your smoothie and adjust the flavor to your preferences. Is there too much strawberry? Is there not enough chocolate? Is the smoothie too tart because you used Greek yogurt instead of regular yogurt? Adjust the flavors just like you would do anything else.

4. Serve in a glass, preferably with a large diameter straw. Garnish if desired.

In closing, feel free to play around with the following smoothie recipes. Don't be afraid to search out other recipes online and try them out. The smoothie recipes in this book are only a frame of reference and starting point for you to begin. Enjoy!

BANANA SMOOTHIE

Ingredients

¼ c. milk
1 c. honey Greek yogurt
4 ripe bananas
2 tbsp. sugar
½ c. ice

BANANAS FOSTER SMOOTHIE

Ingredients

¼ c. milk
1 c. honey Greek yogurt
4 ripe bananas
2 tbsp. maple syrup
2 tsp. cinnamon
2 tbsp. sugar
½ c. ice

BLUEBERRY LEMON SMOOTHIE

Ingredients

1 c. vanilla Greek yogurt
½ c. frozen blueberries
juice of one lemon

BLUEBERRY PINEAPPLE SMOOTHIE

Ingredients

½ c. honey Greek yogurt
½ c. frozen blueberries
1 c. canned pineapple, chopped
2 tbsp. sugar
½ c. ice cubes

CHOCOLATE PEANUT BUTTER BANANA SHAKE

Ingredients

1 scoop chocolate protein powder
¼ c. creamy peanut butter
¼ c. milk
½ c. honey Greek yogurt
2 ripe bananas
1 tbsp. sugar
½ c. ice cubes

MAI TAI SMOOTHIE

Ingredients

1 c. honey Greek yogurt

1 c. canned pineapple, cubed

2 seedless oranges, peeled

4 maraschino cherries or 4 fresh seedless cherries and 2 tbsp. grenadine

¼ c. sugar

½ c. ice

MANGO CHERRY SMOOTHIE

Ingredients

½ c. honey Greek yogurt

1 mango, peeled

8 cherries, seeds and stems removed

¼ c. orange juice

½ c. sugar

STRAWBERRY SMOOTHIE

Ingredients

¼ c. milk

1 c. honey Greek yogurt

2 c. frozen strawberries

2 tbsp. sugar

½ c. ice

STRAWBERRY BANANA SMOOTHIE

Ingredients

1 scoop chocolate protein powder

½ c. milk

¼ c. of honey vanilla Greek yogurt

5 frozen strawberries

1 ripe banana

2 tbsp. sugar

½ c. ice cubes

STRAWBERRY MANGO SMOOTHIE

Ingredients

1 c. honey Greek yogurt

1 c. frozen strawberries

1 mango

½ c. sugar

Recipe Name	Date and Time Eaten	Rating
Recipe Source		Est. Calories

Ingredients and Seasonings

Describe the Taste?

What did you Like?

What did you NOT Like?

What can you add or subtract?

Describe the Texture	Describe the Smell
Any Complications?	How did this recipe make you feel?

Additional Tasting Notes

Recipe Name	Date and Time Eaten	Rating
Recipe Source		Est. Calories

Ingredients and Seasonings

Describe the Taste?

What did you Like?

What did you NOT Like?

What can you add or subtract?

Describe the Texture	Describe the Smell
Any Complications?	How did this recipe make you feel?

Additional Tasting Notes

Recipe Name	Date and Time Eaten	Rating
Recipe Source		Est. Calories

Ingredients and Seasonings

Describe the Taste?

What did you Like?

What did you NOT Like?

What can you add or subtract?

Describe the Texture	Describe the Smell
Any Complications?	How did this recipe make you feel?

Additional Tasting Notes

Recipe Name	Date and Time Eaten	Rating
Recipe Source		Est. Calories

Ingredients and Seasonings

Describe the Taste?

What did you Like?

What did you NOT Like?

What can you add or subtract?

Describe the Texture	Describe the Smell
Any Complications?	How did this recipe make you feel?

Additional Tasting Notes

Recipe Name	Date and Time Eaten	Rating
Recipe Source		Est. Calories

Ingredients and Seasonings

Describe the Taste?

What did you Like?

What did you NOT Like?

What can you add or subtract?

Describe the Texture	Describe the Smell
Any Complications?	How did this recipe make you feel?

Additional Tasting Notes

SAUCE RECIPES

MARINARA (HOME-STYLE)

Recipe Description
A classic marinara sauce made with approval from my wife's Sicilian family. Savory and aromatic with sweetness to balance out the acidity of the natural tomatoes.

Tasting Guidelines
Taste is savory, sweet, and aromatic.
Weight is light, but can be balanced with sugar.
Texture is saucy.
Good for people with low to severe treatment side effects.
Emotional response of home cooked goodness.
Best categorized as classic Italian fare.

Ingredients
2 large cans tomatoes, diced
1 tbsp. olive oil

Flavor Balancers
kosher salt to taste
2 c. Chianti *(red wine)*
black pepper to taste
2 firm shakes of red pepper flakes
2 tbsp. red wine vinegar
¼ c. sugar

Aromatics
2 tbsp. garlic, minced
½ tbsp. oregano
fresh basil *(optional and added at the end)*

Recipe Directions
Take a 2 qt. sauce pan and bring to medium heat. Sauté the garlic in the olive oil until lightly brown. Immediately add oregano, red pepper, and red wine to stop the garlic from processing any further. Allow wine to reduce for 10 minutes. Add salt, black pepper, red wine vinegar, and tomatoes. Stir well. Allow to simmer over medium heat uncovered for 45 minutes to an hour, stirring frequently to avoid burning. After 45 minutes, take a whisk and using a whisking/mashing motion break down the tomatoes until it begins to look more like marinara sauce.

As you break down the tomato chunks, they will mix with the tomato juice and will naturally thicken the sauce. Add sugar and allow to simmer 15 more minutes. Now, we begin the final seasoning process. Add more salt, sugar, and black pepper as necessary. If sauce is acidic and makes the back of your tongue or mouth feel dry, add sugar in small increments. Stir the sauce thoroughly to melt the sugar into the sauce. For a rustic or home-style marinara, whisking should be sufficient to attain the desired consistency. If a more commercial-looking sauce is desired, blend the diced tomatoes in a blender before adding them to the pot.

Chef Tips

You never want your marinara to be bright red. Any marinara sauce that is bright red has not been cooked for long enough for the truly savory aspects of the tomatoes to be released. Therefore, you look for a deeper red similar to a burgundy to tell that the sauce is truly finished. Never, ever, ever, ever cook your marinara sauce over high heat. Plain and simply, you will burn it! Slow and low is the tempo. It is better to slowly prepare your marinara than to burn it.

You also need to make certain that you have a nice, thick-bottomed pot. A thin pot will absolutely burn the sauce before the top of your sauce even gets warm. If you are terrified of burning the sauce, you can always make it in a slow cooker on low heat and let it work over night.

MARSALA WINE SAUCE

Recipe Description
A classic Italian sauce made from butter, mushrooms, chicken stock, and a unique wine. Done correctly, this sauce is savory, sweet, and very rich. It pairs well with most anything. When paired with the pork or chicken scaloppine, it becomes the key ingredient in making chicken or pork marsala. It is especially good on mashed potatoes as well.

Tasting Guidelines
Taste is savory, sweet, and rich.
Weight is medium, but can be balanced vinegar or lemon juice.
Texture is soft and saucy.
Good for people with low to moderate treatment side effects.
Emotional response of delicious Italian food.
Best categorized as classic Italian fare.

Ingredients
8 oz. portabella mushrooms, finely chopped
32 oz. chicken stock
1 stick butter
flour

Flavor Balancers
1 tsp. kosher salt
1–2 c. Marsala wine
2 tsp. black pepper
2 tsp. red pepper
2 tbsp. red wine vinegar
sugar as needed

Aromatics
2 tbsp. garlic, minced
2 tsp. oregano
2 tsp. rosemary
1 tsp. thyme

Recipe Directions
In a large sauté pan, melt the butter at medium heat. Add mushrooms and garlic. Sauté until mushrooms are thoroughly cooked and have almost dissolved into mush. Add oregano, rosemary, thyme, black pepper, and red pepper. Increase heat to a high heat, quickly stir in flour until butter is absorbed. Immediately add wine and deglaze the pan, stirring thoroughly and quickly. Allow the wine to reduce to a thin sauce. Add vinegar and chicken stock, stirring well.

Reduce heat to medium-heat. Allow to work uncovered at least 45 minutes, tasting often. If your sauce is not naturally sweet, you have gotten a bad batch of wine and will need to add sugar to compensate. The sauce should be lightly sweet, very savory, and aromatic. Serve over scaloppine, with your preference of sides. I like mashed potatoes, broccoli, and crusty bread.

ORANGE SAUCE

Recipe Description
A sweet and savory sauce. Perfect over grilled, roasted, and fried meats.

Tasting Guidelines
Taste is sweet and savory.
Weight is light, but can be balanced with sugar.
Texture is soft and saucy.
Good for people with low to moderate treatment side effects.
Emotional response of a fun, sweet citrus-y sauce.
Best categorized as Mediterranean/Chinese fusion.

Ingredients
2 oranges

Flavor Balancers
kosher salt to taste
2 tbsp. light soy sauce
1 tbsp. dark soy sauce
black pepper to taste
2 tsp. red pepper flakes
1 tbsp. red wine vinegar
1 c. orange juice
1 c. sugar

Aromatics
1 tsp. ground ginger

Recipe Directions
In a medium sauce pan, combine orange juice, red pepper flakes, dark and light soy sauce, red wine vinegar, and ginger. Bring to a medium heat. Allow to simmer 10 minutes. Take one orange and cut in half. Squeeze fresh juice into sauce, taking care to strain the seeds. Place orange rind into sauce. Allow to simmer 10 additional minutes.

Remove rind. Slowly whisk in sugar. Taste for sweetness. Serve with fresh orange slices as garnish.

Chef Tips
This sauce is wonderful over roasted pork loin or chicken breasts. It is also suitable for use in the classic Chinese dishes orange chicken, orange beef, and orange pork.

PESTO

Recipe Description
A northern Italian favorite. A simple sauce made from basil leaves. It is incredibly versatile and can be placed on anything that is of a lighter weight. Especially good with chicken. Pesto was huge in the '80s and '90s, which was captured in the iconic sitcom Seinfeld where George (paraphrased) says, "Ya know? I just don't care for pesto."

Tasting Guidelines
Taste is clean.
Weight is light, but can be balanced with parmesan.
Texture is soft and saucy.
Good for people with low to severe treatment side effects.
Emotional response of feeling clean and refreshed.
Best categorized as northern Italian.

Ingredients
1 lb. fresh basil leaves
½ c. extra virgin olive oil
½ c. parmesan
2 tbsp. pine nuts *(optional)*
2 tbsp. garlic, minced *(optional)*

Recipe Directions
Place basil, garlic, parmesan, and pine nuts into blender. Pulse the blender until basil is finely chopped. Add olive oil until it forms a saucy consistency. May require more olive oil than the recipe calls for.

Chef Tips
Pesto is actually a real nice, light sauce. It has tons of uses. You can put it on pasta, sandwiches, toast, brush it on chicken, and even substitute it in any recipe that fresh basil is required. For example, in caprese salad, you can substitute pesto instead of fresh basil leaves and toss with balsamic vinegar instead of red wine vinaigrette for a change of pace.

PLUM SAUCE

Recipe Description
A classic Spanish sauce. Mostly unheard of in the United States. The sauce is sweet, tangy, and savory. The best way to describe this sauce is that it is like a Spanish barbecue sauce. The dried plums take care of the consistency and thickness of the sauce, eliminating the need for a thickener. The dried plums are also great for digestion. This is an added benefit as chemotherapy can cause problems in this area. Use this sauce over grilled foods for best results.

Tasting Guidelines
Taste is savory and sweet.
Weight is medium, but can be balanced with savory and sweet.
Texture is soft and saucy.
Good for people with low to moderate treatment side effects.
Emotional response of eating a tasty barbecue sauce.
Best categorized as classic Spanish.

Ingredients
8 oz. pitted prunes (*dried plums*)
1 c. water

Aromatics
1 sprig of rosemary
1 tsp. cinnamon

Flavor Balancers
1 tsp. kosher salt
½ c. red wine or sherry
2 tsp. freshly ground black pepper
1 tbsp. red wine vinegar
1 tbsp. sugar

Recipe Directions
In a medium sauce pan, combine the prunes, cinnamon, salt, black pepper, red wine, rosemary, and water. Bring to a boil until prunes have re-hydrated. Then, using a whisk, mash the prunes until they have become more liquefied and mix well. Add one tbsp. of red wine vinegar and sugar. Whisk well and allow to simmer for 5–10 minutes. Taste sauce and adjust seasonings as necessary. Sauce should taste like savory sugared plums with a bit of dryness on the back.

Chef Tips
This sauce is amazing! Prunes are also packed with potassium, B12, B6, fiber, and an enzyme that helps re-hydrate your intestines. This makes it easier to go to the bathroom. Don't be afraid of this sauce because of the prunes. The added sugar and cinnamon really livens it up. And, you will be glad you ate this! This recipe is also great for people who are getting backed up and bloated. This sauce is a great all natural way to help get things moving along. *Wink*

TZATZIKI SAUCE

Recipe Description
A classic Greek yogurt sauce typically associated with gyro sandwiches. This recipe is fabulous not just on sandwiches, but also served on bread, pitas, or over a salad as a dressing. The versatility of this sauce is amazing. Given its yogurt-based construction, you would assume it is heavy when in fact it is very light.

Tasting Guidelines
Taste is savory, sweet, and tangy.
Weight is light, but can be balanced with honey.
Texture is soft and creamy.
Good for people with low to severe treatment side effects.
Emotional response of unexpected yumminess.
Best categorized as Greek.

Ingredients
1 large tub honeyed Greek yogurt
1 large cucumber, peeled and diced
3 Roma tomatoes, diced
½ medium sized red onion, diced

Garnish
crusty break or pita bread to serve

Flavor Balancers
kosher salt to taste
black pepper to taste
¼ c. red wine vinaigrette dressing

Aromatics
1 tbsp. garlic, minced

Recipe Directions
Take diced cucumber, tomatoes, and red onion and place in a large mixing bowl. Shake red wine vinaigrette dressing well and coat thoroughly. Sprinkle in salt, pepper, and garlic. Allow to marinate at room temperature at least one hour or in the refrigerator for two hours, stirring frequently. Mix in yogurt. Toss gently. Allow to marinate in refrigerator until flavors become cohesive.

Chef Tips
The longer the flavors have to sit together the more cohesive they become. If flavors do not emphasize the sweetness, stir in honey until you reach desired sweetness. Serve with fresh pitas or fresh bread. It also makes a fantastic dressing for salads and can be eaten as a condiment over falafel, gyros, other sandwiches, just eaten by itself, or over oatmeal. If mouth sores are problematic, you can puree the cucumber, onions, and tomatoes for a much softer texture.

Recipe Name	Date and Time Eaten	Rating

Recipe Source	Est. Calories

Ingredients and Seasonings

Describe the Taste?

What did you Like?

What did you NOT Like?

What can you add or subtract?

Describe the Texture	Describe the Smell

Any Complications?	How did this recipe make you feel?

Additional Tasting Notes

Recipe Name	Date and Time Eaten	Rating
Recipe Source		Est. Calories

Ingredients and Seasonings

Describe the Taste?

What did you Like?

What did you NOT Like?

What can you add or subtract?

Describe the Texture	Describe the Smell
Any Complications?	How did this recipe make you feel?

Additional Tasting Notes

Recipe Name	Date and Time Eaten	Rating

Recipe Source	Est. Calories

Ingredients and Seasonings

Describe the Taste?

What did you Like?

What did you NOT Like?

What can you add or subtract?

Describe the Texture	Describe the Smell

Any Complications?	How did this recipe make you feel?

Additional Tasting Notes

Recipe Name	Date and Time Eaten	Rating
Recipe Source		Est. Calories

Ingredients and Seasonings

Describe the Taste?

What did you Like?

What did you NOT Like?

What can you add or subtract?

Describe the Texture	Describe the Smell
Any Complications?	How did this recipe make you feel?

Additional Tasting Notes

SUPPLEMENTAL INFORMATION

STANDARD TO METRIC MEASUREMENT CONVERSION CHARTS AND INFORMATION

These are some handy charts for referencing different measurements. This so that you can increase your recipes, decrease your recipes, or convert them to metric if you do not use USA standard measurements. Converting recipes is actually very easy once you understand the basics of measurement. American recipes use fluid measurements for most household recipes, even for dry ingredients. As opposed to metric based recipes which tend to use weight of ingredients. If you live outside of the United States, you can always pick up a set of American measuring cups and measuring spoons off of *amazon.com* for your convenience. Once you learn to cook with American measurements, you'll find that our old-fashioned way is actually very organic and easy to use!

Fluid Measurements

Standard Name	Abbreviations	Milliliters	Ounces *(Fluid)*	Components
1 teaspoon	t., tsp., tsps.	5ml	.1667 ounces	none
1 tablespoon	T., tbsp.	15 ml	.5 ounces	3 teaspoons
1 cup	c, cp.	240 ml	8 ounces	16 tablespoons
1 pint	p., pt.	480 ml	16 ounces	2 cups
1 quart	q., qt.	960 ml	32 ounces	2 pints
1 gallon	g., gal.	3840 ml	128 ounces	4 quarts

Weight Measurements

Standard Name	Abbreviations	Converted	Components
1 ounce	o., oz.	28.35 grams	none
1 pound	lb., lbs., #	453.59 grams	16 ounces
1 gram	g., gm.	0.035 ounces	1000 milligrams
1 kilogram	kg.	2.2 pounds	1000 grams

Temperature Measurements

Fahrenheit	Celsius	Significance of Temperature
0	-18	long term freezer storage
32	0	freezing water
40	5	refrigerator temperature
145	63	seafood and veggies cooked, ready to eat food temperature
155	69	beef, and red meats well-done temperature

165	74	chicken, turkey, poultry well-done temperature
212	100	boiling water
300	149	low bake temperature
350	177	medium bake temperature
375	191	medium-high bake temperature
400	205	high bake temperature
425	219	roasting temperature
450	233	high roasting temperature

These temperatures are the direct conversions from Fahrenheit to Celsius. Feel free to convert them into easier to use versions that are more appropriate to your region.

Specialty Measurements

1 pinch is the amount of seasoning you can pick up between your thumb and forefinger.
1 dash is roughly equivalent to 3 pinches.
1 stick of butter = 4 ounces or 113.34 grams. In the US, butter is sold by the pound.
But, each pound is broken up into long thin quarters that we call "sticks."
1 cup of flour weighs 120 grams when measured correctly.

BRITISH ENGLISH TO AMERICAN ENGLISH CONCEPT CONVERSION CHART

Because the English speaking world is spread across many continents with local variations at each turn, I have provided the following concept conversion chart. Hopefully, this concept conversion chart can help my international readers understand what each ingredient is! This should also help anyone who wants to use recipes from other English speaking countries.

American English	British English
All-Purpose Flour	Plain Flour
Aluminum Foil	Tin Foil
Bacon	Streaky Bacon
Bell Peppers	Green/Red Peppers
Blender	Liquidizer
Broiler	Grill
Candied Fruits	Glace Fruits
Canned	Tinned
Chili	Chili Con Carne
Chips	Crisps
Chop	Cutlet
Cilantro	Fresh Coriander Leaves
Corn	Sweet Corn/Maize
Corn Starch	Cornflour
Eggplant	Aubergine
Entree	Main Course
Fava Bean	Broad Bean
Filet Mignon or Tenderloin	Fillet Steak
Flatware or Silverware	Cutlery
French Fries	Chips
Green Onions	Spring Onions
Ground Meat	Minced Meat
Half and Half	Single Cream
Ham	Gammon
Hard Cider	Cider
Heavy Cream	Double Cream
Hot Sauce	Chili Sauce

Jelly	Jam
Light Brown Cane Sugar	Demerara Sugar
Oatmeal, Cooked	Porridge
Pit	Stone
Plastic Wrap	Clingfilm
Porter House	Sirloin
Pot Pie	Pie
Preserves	Conserves
Romaine Lettuce	Cos Lettuce
Sausage *(Breakfast)*	Banger
Self-Rising Flour	Self-Raising Flour
Shuck	Hull
Sirloin	Rump Steak
Skillet	Frying Pan
Small Shrimp	Prawn
Snow Peas	Mangetout
Soda, Pop, Soda Pop, Coke	Soft Drink, Pop, Fizzy Juice
String Beans or Green Beans	French Beans
Wax Paper	Greaseproof Paper
Whole-Wheat Flour	Wholemeal Flour
Zucchini or Summer Squash	Courgette

HERBS AND SPICES CHART

Flavor, Function, When to add them, and Common Uses

Herb/Spice	Flavor/ Function	Common Uses
Anise *(Spice)*	**Flavor:** Licorice flavor **Function:** Warming. Add in beginning of a dish.	Mediterranean cuisine, Middle Eastern cuisine, Chinese cuisine, Indian cuisine, Vietnamese cuisine, fish, cakes, cookies, breads, stews
Allspice *(Spice)*	**Flavor:** Pepper with notes of cinnamon, nutmeg, and cloves. **Function:** Rounded, spiced flavor. Add in the beginning of a dish.	beef, chicken, curries, fruits, ginger, Jamaican cuisine, meats, pumpkin, squash
Basil *(Herb)*	**Flavor:** Sweet with a hint of licorice. **Function:** Adds freshness to a dish. Add at the very end of a dish. Absolutely last.	bell peppers, cheese, chicken, eggplant, eggs, fish, garlic, Italian cuisine, lamb, lemon, meats, Mediterranean cuisine, mint, olive oil, oregano, pasta, pesto, pizza, salads, salmon, salt, shellfish, soups, Thai cuisine, tomatoes, tomato sauces, vegetables, vinegar, watermelon, zucchini
Bay Leaves *(Herb)*	**Flavor:** Sweet **Function:** Adds richness and savory to dishes. Add in the beginning to give time to work throughout the dish.	beans, fish, meats, parsley, rice, soups, stews, stocks and broths, thyme, tomatoes and tomato sauces
Caraway Seeds *(Spice)*	**Flavor:** Sweet, sour **Function:** Adds zest. Add at the beginning of dish or baking.	breads *(esp. pumpernickel and rye)*, cheese, German cuisine, pork, potatoes, sauerkraut
Cardamom *(Spice)*	**Flavor:** Sweet, pungent **Function:** Adds heating effect. Add at the beginning of a dish.	chicken, cinnamon, coffee, coriander, curries, dates, desserts, ginger, Indian cuisine, lamb, oranges, rice, tea
Cayenne Pepper *(Spice)*	**Flavor:** Spicy **Function:** Adds spiciness to a dish. Add at the beginning of a dish.	bell peppers, Cajun cuisine, fish, tomatoes

Chives *(Herb)*	**Flavor:** Green onion **Function:** Adds light onion flavor to dishes. Added at the end.	cheese, eggs, parsley, pork, potatoes, salads, sauces, soups, sour cream, tarragon, vegetables
Cilantro *(Fresh Coriander Leaves) (Herb)*	**Flavor:** Sweet, sour, citrus **Function:** Adds a cooling note to spicy dishes and a freshness to dishes. Add at the very end. Mostly used as a garnish.	Asian cuisines, avocados, chicken, chili peppers, coconut, cumin, curries, fish, garlic, ginger, Indian cuisine, lemon, lemongrass, lime, Mexican cuisine, mint, rice, salads, salsas, tacos, Thai cuisine, tomatoes, yogurt
Cinnamon *(Spice)*	**Flavor:** Sweet, bitter, pungent **Function:** Adds warmth to dishes. Add in the beginning of a dish. Needs time to work in and mellow.	apples, baked dishes and goods, bananas, hot beverages, blueberries, breakfast/brunch, chicken, chocolate, coffee, cloves, curries, custards, desserts, fruits, ginger, lamb, lemon, Mexican cuisine, Middle Eastern cuisine, Moroccan cuisine, mulled wine nutmeg, oranges, pears, pecans, pork, rice, sugar, tea, vanilla
Cloves *(Spice)*	**Flavor:** Sweet, pungent **Function:** Adds warmth to dishes. Add in the beginning of a dish.	apples, chocolate, cinnamon, ginger, ham, lemon, mulled wine, oranges, pork
Coriander *(Spice)*	**Flavor:** Sour, pungent, dry **Function:** Cools dish's flavors. Add in the middle of cooking a dish.	chicken, chili peppers, citrus, crab, cumin, curries, fish, garlic, lentils, pepper, pork
Cumin *(Spice)*	**Flavor:** Bitter, sweet **Function:** Heating of dishes. Add in the middle of cooking a dish or early if used in a marinade. It needs time to de-funk.	beans, chickpeas, coriander, couscous, curries, eggplant, garlic, Indian cuisine, lamb, lentils, Mexican cuisine, Moroccan cuisine, pork, potatoes, rice, sausages, tomatoes
Curry Powder *(Spice Blend)*	**Flavor:** Bittersweet, pungent **Function:** Adds aromatic quality to dishes. Add early to a dish. Needs time to mellow.	ginger, Indian cuisine, Thai cuisine, vegetables

Dill *(Herb)*	**Flavor:** Sour, sweet **Function:** Adds freshness to dishes. Add at the very end of a dish. It is a delicate herb.	beets, cabbage, carrots, cilantro, cucumbers, eggs, fish, parsley, pickles, potatoes, salads, salmon
Fennel *(Spice)*	**Flavor:** Sweet **Function:** It adds a licorice sweetness to dishes. Add midway through cooking a dish.	Chinese cuisine, fish, five spice powder, Italian cuisine, pork, sausages, shellfish
Garlic *(Root Vegetable)*	**Flavor:** Aromatic, touch of spicy **Function:** Adds warmth to dishes. Always add the very beginning of a dish. **Chef's Note:** There are very few applications that cannot be benefited by the addition of garlic.	basil, cheese, chicken, Chinese cuisine, French cuisine, Indian cuisine, Italian cuisine, Korean cuisine, lamb, lemon, meats, Mediterranean cuisine, Mexican cuisine, Middle Eastern cuisine, Moroccan cuisine, mushrooms, mustard, olive oil, onions, salt, tomatoes, Vietnamese cuisine, vinegars
Ginger *(Spice)*	**Flavor:** Sour and hot **Function:** Adds warmth to dishes. **Chef's Note:** Add at the beginning of a dish if you want it to mellow. Add towards the end if you want it to add a pop of flavor.	apples, Asian cuisine, basil, beverages
Marjoram *(Herb)*	**Flavor:** Sweet and spicy and in the same family as oregano, just lighter in flavor. **Function:** Adds a light, crisp pepperiness. Add in the middle of a dish.	basil, cheese-goat mozzarella, Italian Cuisine, Greek Cuisine

Mint *(Herb)*	**Flavor:** Sweet crisp herb **Function:** It adds a subtle, cleansing pop. Like basil add at end of cooking so you don't lose its pop. **Chef's Note:** Add at the very end of a dish. The flavor is very delicate.	beverages, chocolate, cream, ice cream, desserts, teas
Nutmeg *(Spice)*	**Flavor:** Aromatic spice. Typically used in fall and winter dishes. **Function:** To add a sense of warmth to a dish. Add to food in the beginning. If adding to drinks, add at the end as a topper.	apples, cheese, chicken, cream/milk, desserts, eggnog, lamb, pasta and pasta sauces, puddings, pumpkin, rice, veal
Oregano *(Herb)*	**Flavor:** Rich, aromatic, and peppery herb. **Function:** It adds a nice, subtle black pepper flavor that blends well with food. Add at the beginning of a dish to give it time to work through the dish.	beans, beef, chicken, fish, lamb, meats, pasta and pasta sauces, salads, soups
Paprika *(Spice)*	**Flavor:** Sweet-hot, depending on variety. **Function:** It adds a very light touch of warmth and heat. Due to its muted and subtle flavor, it is mainly used to add color to a dish. Add at the very end.	beef, chicken, eggs, fish, pork

Parsley (*Herb*)	**Flavor:** Bitter and fresh **Function:** To be used as a pallet cleanser. Add at the very end. Always put on top. You never want to cook it into a dish. **Chef's Note:** Flat leaf aka Italian parsley is fantastic to use in dishes where you need a freshness and a crispness. Parsley is also fantastic for cleansing palates.	basil, carrots, chicken, eggplant, fish, pasta and pasta sauces, pork, potatoes, soups, stews, stocks, vegetables
Pepper, Black (*Spice*)	**Flavor:** Mildly spicy and warm **Function:** The most basic spice to fill out a flavor profile. Add in the beginning of a dish.	beef, eggs, game, meats/red, salt, steaks
Poppy Seeds (*Spice*)	**Flavor:** Sweet and aromatic **Function:** Used mainly in baked goods to add a fun floral aroma. Usually added before baking baked goods.	breads, cakes, cookies, butter, cheese, pasta, potatoes, salads and salad dressings, zucchini
Red Pepper (*Spice*)	**Flavor:** Spicy **Function:** Adds spiciness and heat to a dish. Add in small increments in the beginning of a dish.	meats, seafood, any meal that you want to have a spicy kick
Rosemary (*Herb*)	**Flavor:** Aromatic herb **Function:** Add early in cooking to add a rich warmth and depth to your dishes.	beans, breads, butter, chicken, duck, fish, lamb
Sage (*Herb*)	**Flavor:** Highly aromatic. It is the single ingredient that makes everything it is in smell like Thanksgiving. **Function:** Add last in cooking to add warmth and depth to the dish.	stuffing, turkey, poultry, traditional American food

Savory *(Herb)*	**Flavor:** Savory is exactly like it sounds, savory. Its flavor is a blend between thyme, rosemary, and sage. **Function:** It adds savoriness and aromatic quality to a dish. Add early in cooking.	beans, beef, chicken, garlic, red meat, starchy potatoes, tomatoes
Tarragon *(Herb)*	**Flavor:** Liquorice flavor, heavier than basil but lighter than normal liquorice flavor. **Function:** It adds lightness and freshness to a dish. Add last to a dish.	acidic foods, poultry, eggs, fish, light flavored dishes
Thyme *(Herb)*	**Flavor:** Aromatic and rich **Function:** Adds warmth to dishes and gives food a wholesome taste. Add about midway through the dish.	marinara sauce, tomatoes, red meats, poultry, roasted meats, starchy vegetables
Turmeric *(Spice)*	**Flavor:** It's the main spice in curry. It is the spice that gives seasoned salt its flavor. **Function:** Warms up a dish. Add in the beginning or middle of cooking a dish.	chicken, curries, Indian cuisine, Middle Eastern cuisine, Moroccan cuisine, pork, rice, Thai cuisine

REFERENCE PAGE

A special thanks to the following resources that I referenced while doing research for *Cooking for Chemo... and After!* These are all great resources. I highly encourage reading of the source material for an even greater understanding of culinary theory and applicable material.

Books:

The Complete Mediterranean Cookbook
By Tess Mallos

The Flavor Bible
By Karen Page and Andrew Bornenburg

The Wok
A Complete and Easy Guide to Preparing a Wide Variety of Authentic Chinese Favorites.
By Gary Lee

On Cooking
A Textbook of Culinary Fundamentals
By Sarah R. Labensky and Alan M. Hause

Joy of Cooking
By Rombauer, Becker, Becker

Websites:

usda.gov
smithsonianmag.com
blogs.scientificamerican.com
health.harvard.edu
sciencedirect.com
m.ajcn.nutrition.org
medicinenet.com
mayoclinic.org

CONNECT WITH US

Website
www.cookingforchemo.org
www.chefryancallahan.com
www.callahanpublishing.com

Instagram
@chef_ryan_callahan

Twitter
@cookingforchemo

Facebook
facebook.com/cookingforchemo

Pinterest
pinterest.com/cookingforchemo

ABOUT THE AUTHOR

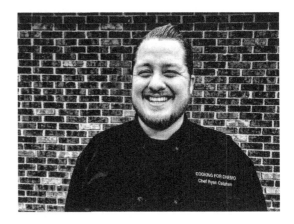

Chef Ryan Callahan is an award winning author and chef. He is the author of *Chef Ryan's How-to-Cook Cookbook, Cooking for Chemo ...and After!, Cooking for Kids with Cancer,* and *Chef Ryan Callahan's Tasting Journal.*

Chef Ryan has won two Gourmand World Cookbook Awards for his culinary expertise.

2016 Gourmand World Cookbook Award Winner: Best New Health and Nutrition Cookbook, USA; for his ground-breaking book, *Cooking for Chemo ...and After!*

2018 Gourmand World Cookbook Award Winner: Most Innovative Cookbook, USA; for *Chef Ryan's How-to-Cook Cookbook*

Chef Ryan Callahan is a hospitality industry veteran with over 15 years of hands-on culinary experience in the kitchen and front of house. When Chef Ryan isn't working on his own projects, he works as a freelance culinary consultant specializing in commercial product and recipe development.

Made in the USA
Monee, IL
28 August 2021